Non-Surgical Rhinoplasty

Plastic surgeons specializing in rhinoplasty will here find an essential resource bringing together the expertise they will need to offer non-invasive techniques in their practice.

- Brings together all a surgeon needs to know for safe and effective non-invasive rhinoplasty
- Offers a one-stop resource for surgeons wishing to add injection techniques to their practice
- Presents a masterclass from world experts

Non-Surgical Rhinoplasty is the second title of a series to be published in partnership with *PRIME* Journal and the Aesthetic Multispecialty Society (AMS). The first title was Ali Pirayesh, Dario Bertossi, Izolda Heydenrych, eds, *Aesthetic Facial Anatomy Essentials for Injections*, 2020.

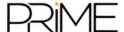

PRIME Journal is the leading authority on aesthetic and anti-aging medicine, providing industry news, insightful analysis, and key data, as well as the most high-quality research articles in the market. It's because of this that *PRIME* attracts leading authors who provide authoritative analysis on the issues that matter most to the industry. The aesthetic and anti-aging industry is a global one and deserves a dedicated international publication—a voice that will not only communicate, but educate, motivate, and inspire you with the latest, most applicable and usable information you need to do your work smarter, better, and more effectively. Published both in print and online, *PRIME* is an essential tool for physicians, surgeons, dermatologists, and practitioners alike.

If you have not already subscribed to *PRIME*, visit the website today at www.prime-journal.com to guarantee each issue of the journal is delivered to your work or home.

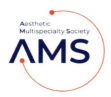

The Aesthetic Multispecialty Society (AMS) was created to gather the Aesthetic Medical community together, promoting education and knowledge sharing with the primary goal of improving techniques and good practice in the field of Aesthetic Dermatology and Surgery. The Aesthetic Multispecialty Society provides an advanced comprehensive platform created for all practitioners of Aesthetic Surgery and Aesthetic and Anti-aging medicine.

All our features have been designed to bring our members closer together and create a society that puts Aesthetic Medicine at the heart of everything we do. Benefits of joining the Aesthetic Multispecialty Society include:

- AMS membership certificate
- Special discounted rates on many international events
- Attend live webinars or watch on demand at your convenience
- Access to educational videos and workshops from major aesthetic medicine events
- Access to online forum discussions with your peers
- Discounted rates on scientific books and journals
- Priority to submit your article in *PRIME* Journal
- Priority to apply to be a speaker at an AMS-affiliated congress and/or educational training course worldwide

*Listing in the AMS directory of aesthetic and/or anti-aging professionals
*Receive the AMS newsletter with updates on the market products, scientific articles, and events

The AMS Scientific Committee is composed of core and recognized experts who have contributed over many years to the education of thousands of doctors through university programs, seminars and conferences across the globe. The AMS is highly engaged with many of the leading international events in the sector including AMWC Monaco, ICAD, FACE, Vegas Cosmetic Surgery & Aesthetic Dermatology (VCS), Miami Cosmetic Surgery (MCS), The Aesthetic Show (TAS), and many other educational and training programs, including the CFA and VISAGE University Certification programs. Please visit the website at https://multispecialtysociety.com.

Non-Surgical Rhinoplasty

Edited by

Dario Bertossi, MD

Associate Professor of Maxillofacial Surgery, Specialist in Maxillofacial Surgery, Otolaryngology, Facial Plastic Surgeon, Head and Neck Department, Department of Surgery, Dentistry, Pediatrics and Gynaecology, University of Verona, Verona, Italy; and Professor of Practice, University of London Centre for Integrated Medical and Translational Research, London, UK

Riccardo Nocini, MD

Resident in Otorhinolaryngology, Head and Neck Department, University of Verona, Verona, Italy

Ali Pirayesh, MD, FCC (Plast)

Plastic, Reconstructive and Aesthetic Surgeon, Founder, Amsterdam Plastic Surgery Clinic, the Netherlands; Consultant, Burns and Tissue Regeneration Unit, University Hospital, Gent, Belgium; and Research Consultant, University College Hospital, London, UK

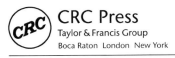

CRC Press is an imprint of the
Taylor & Francis Group, an **informa** business

First edition published 2023
by CRC Press
6000 Broken Sound Parkway NW, Suite 300, Boca Raton, FL 33487–2742

and by CRC Press
4 Park Square, Milton Park, Abingdon, Oxon, OX14 4RN

CRC Press is an imprint of Taylor & Francis Group, LLC

© 2023 selection and editorial matter, Dario Bertossi, Riccardo Nocini, Ali Pirayesh individual chapters, the contributors

This book contains information obtained from authentic and highly regarded sources. While all reasonable efforts have been made to publish reliable data and information, neither the author[s] nor the publisher can accept any legal responsibility or liability for any errors or omissions that may be made. The publishers wish to make clear that any views or opinions expressed in this book by individual editors, authors or contributors are personal to them and do not necessarily reflect the views/opinions of the publishers. The information or guidance contained in this book is intended for use by medical, scientific or health-care professionals and is provided strictly as a supplement to the medical or other professional's own judgement, their knowledge of the patient's medical history, relevant manufacturer's instructions and the appropriate best practice guidelines. Because of the rapid advances in medical science, any information or advice on dosages, procedures or diagnoses should be independently verified. The reader is strongly urged to consult the relevant national drug formulary and the drug companies' and device or material manufacturers' printed instructions, and their websites, before administering or utilizing any of the drugs, devices or materials mentioned in this book. This book does not indicate whether a particular treatment is appropriate or suitable for a particular individual. Ultimately it is the sole responsibility of the medical professional to make his or her own professional judgements, so as to advise and treat patients appropriately. The authors and publishers have also attempted to trace the copyright holders of all material reproduced in this publication and apologize to copyright holders if permission to publish in this form has not been obtained. If any copyright material has not been acknowledged please write and let us know so we may rectify in any future reprint.

Except as permitted under U.S. Copyright Law, no part of this book may be reprinted, reproduced, transmitted, or utilized in any form by any electronic, mechanical, or other means, now known or hereafter invented, including photocopying, microfilming, and recording, or in any information storage or retrieval system, without written permission from the publishers.

For permission to photocopy or use material electronically from this work, access www.copyright.com or contact the Copyright Clearance Center, Inc. (CCC), 222 Rosewood Drive, Danvers, MA 01923, 978–750–8400. For works that are not available on CCC please contact mpkbookspermissions@tandf.co.uk

Trademark notice: Product or corporate names may be trademarks or registered trademarks and are used only for identification and explanation without intent to infringe.

ISBN: 978-1-032-30344-4 (hbk)
ISBN: 978-1-032-30345-1 (pbk)
ISBN: 978-1-003-30462-3 (ebk)

DOI: 10.1201/9781003304623

Typeset in Times
by Apex CoVantage, LLC

Access the Support Material: https://resourcecentre.routledge.com/books/9781032303444

Contents

List of Contributors viii

Chapter 1.1
Introduction: The New Era of Nasal Aesthetic Treatments 1
Dario Bertossi, Riccardo Nocini, and Ali Pirayesh

Chapter 1.2
Hyaluronic Acid Fillers 3
Dario Bertossi, Riccardo Nocini, and Ali Pirayesh

Chapter 1.3
Botulinum Toxin 6
Dario Bertossi, Riccardo Nocini, and Ali Pirayesh

Chapter 1.4
Combined Devices 8
Dario Bertossi and Salvatore Chirumbolo

Chapter 1.5
The HA Filler Market 10
Dario Bertossi, Riccardo Nocini, and Ali Pirayesh

Chapter 1.6
The Botulinum Toxin Market 12
Dario Bertossi, Riccardo Nocini, and Ali Pirayesh

Chapter 1.7
The Impact of Social Networks 13
Dario Bertossi, Riccardo Nocini, and Ali Pirayesh

Chapter 2
Anatomy 17

Chapter 2.1
Surface Anatomy 18
Dario Bertossi and Ali Pirayesh

Chapter 2.2
Deep Anatomy 23
Dario Bertossi, Ali Pirayesh, Riccardo Nocini, and Andrea Sbarbati

Chapter 3
Clinical Aspects 28

Chapter 3.1
Clinical Defects and the Technical Approach 29
Woodrow Wilson and Dario Bertossi

Chapter 3.2
Patient Consultation 39
Dario Bertossi and Ali Pirayesh

Chapter 4
Preoperative Diagnostics 43

Chapter 4.1
Preoperative Diagnosis 44
Fernando Urdiales

Chapter 4.2
Skin Conditions Affecting the Nose and Perinasal Area 50
Izolda Heydenrych

Chapter 4.3
Conditions Affecting the Nose and Perinasal Skin and Their Assessment and Diagnosis 62
Ilaria Proietti

Chapter 5
Surgical Rhinoplasty 72
Dario Bertossi, Enrico Robotti, and Carlos Neves

Chapter 6
Non-Surgical Rhinoplasty 78
Dario Bertossi, Ali Pirayesh, and Alwyn D'Souza

Chapter 7
Surrounding Areas 101
Ash Mohsaebi, Riccardo Nocini, and Ekaterina Gutop

Chapter 8
Non-Surgical Profileplasty 107
Thierry Besins, Ali Pirayesh, and Dario Bertossi

Chapter 9
Complications from Hyaluronic Acid Fillers 112
Koenraad De Boulle

Chapter 10
Clinical Cases from the Experts 121
Introductory Video Section 122
Dario Bertossi

Chapter 10.1
Non-Surgical Rhinoplasty: Long-Term Correction after Five Years 123
Ada Trindade de Almeida

Chapter 10.2
Asian Cases 127
Chris Qiong Li

Chapter 10.3
Clinical Case: Profileplasty 130
Dario Bertossi

Chapter 10.4
Clinical Case: The Slavic Face 134
Ekaterina Gutop

Chapter 10.5
Clinical Case: Rhino 4-Point Technique with Fillers of Different Densities 136
Fernando Silikovich

Chapter 10.6
Clinical Case: Nasofrontal Angle with Ultrasound Correlation 140
Fernando Urdiales

Chapter 10.7
My Tinkerbell Tip Lift Technique 143
K. Kay Durairaj

Chapter 10.8
Clinical Case: Long Duration of HA Fillers in the Nose 146
Per Heden

Chapter 10.9
Clinical Case: Nasal Hump (Multiple Approach) 148
Philippe Magistretti

Chapter 10.10
Clinical Case: Nasal Hump (Dorsum Approach) 150
Rami Abadi

Chapter 10.11
Clinical Case: Rhino-Modeling in South America 151
Raúl Banegas

Index 153

Contributors

Rami Abadi
RA Clinic
Beirut, Lebanon

Raúl Banegas
Banegas Aesthetic Medicine
Buenos Aires, Argentina

Thierry Besins
Clinique Saint-Georges
Nice, France

Salvatore Chirumbolo
Medicine
University of Verona
Verona, Italy

Alwyn D'Souza
University College of London
London UK

Ada Trindade de Almeida
Clinica Dermatologica
Sao Paulo, Brasil

Koenraad De Boulle
Aalst Dermatology Clinic
Aalst Belgium
University College London
London, UK

K. Kay Durairaj
Head & Neck Surgery
Huntington Memorial Hospital
UCLA/Olive View Medical Center
Los Angeles, California

Ekaterina Gutop
Actual Clinic
Yaroslavl, Russia

Per Heden
Karolinska Institute
Stockholm, Sweden

Izolda Heydenrych
Cape Town Cosmetic Sermatology Centre
University of Stellenbosh
Cape Town, South Africa

Chris Qiong Li
Angel Swan Clinic
Shanghai, China

Philippe Magistretti
The Summit Clinic
Crans Montana, Switzerland

Ash Mohsaebi
University College of London
London UK

Carlos Neves
Cardiovascular Consultants of Southern Delaware
Lewes, Delaware

Ilaria Proietti
Sapienza University of Rome
Rome Italy

Enrico Robotti
Clinica Villa Sant'Apollonia
Bergamo, Italy

Andrea Sbarbati
Anatomy and Histology
University of Verona
Verona, Italy

Fernando Silikovich
Estetica Buenos Aires
Buenos Aires, Argentina

Fernando Urdiales
Instituto Médico Miramar
Malaga, Spain

Woodrow Wilson
Clinical Imaging Australia PTY Ltd
Melbourne, Australia

CHAPTER **1.1**

Introduction
The New Era of Nasal Aesthetic Treatments

Dario Bertossi, Riccardo Nocini, and Ali Pirayesh

Facial aesthetics has become a leading factor for social communication, as the human face can be considered the frontline of any relationship skill, leading crucial decisions and moving any individual's attitude in the relation dynamics. Having an "appealing look" has gained the utmost importance in modern life, as the attractiveness of the human face impacts a huge number of daily life aspects [1]. Face affects also several hallmarks of the various cultural habits and beliefs in mankind [2], as it is recognized in many theories on socialization and anthropological evolution, recently reviewed by Langlois et al., as follows: "the effects of facial attractiveness are robust and pandemic, extending beyond initial impressions of strangers to actual interactions with those whom people know and observe" [3, page 404]. To date, the role of the face in the globalized world has achieved a primacy in communication skills, thus moving our conceptual perception of the "face beauty" throughout the rapid evolution of fashion and habits caused by the frequent cross-talks with different cultures and moods, even at the neurophysiological level [4–11]. This has lead, to date, to a huge amount of interests and requests to modify one's own face in order to be better targeted to aesthetic models, usually borrowed from leaders and attractive people in the communication market [12,13].

The concept of beauty, from a neurological point of view, lies alongside the concept of symmetry. The same attractiveness of a face is deeply affected by its symmetry, a harmonious proportion of anatomical parts, collectively sharing the concept of what represents an "ideal" face [14–19]. In this context, some facial anatomical regions are particularly crucial; a leading role is exerted, for example, by the nose with its relationship with overall face and the profile.

Requests to fit the nose to an ideal symmetry or adjust, refine or correct imperfections are increasing hugely in the real world to date, particularly with non-surgical rhinoplasty [20,21].

Any individualized strategy for rhinoplasty, septoplasty or facial profileplasty or other approaches collectively gathered in the term "facelift", may be critical to achieve a full-face aesthetic view, particularly if addressing a rejuvenating process. The enormous availability and affordability of non-surgical practices in facial aesthetics worldwide has generated a huge market of nasal aesthetic treatments, enhanced by the concurrent, quite paroxysmal, query to have an attractive look.

Global market research studies have forecasted that the rhinoplasty market will be worth over 2 billion dollars in 2027, most of which will be in non-surgical rhinoplasty. The size of the rhinoplasty implants market has been valued at 700 million dollars in 2020 and is expected to grow at a compound annual growth rate (CAGR) of 15.9% between 2021 and 2027, despite the complex networks of queries/offerings worldwide, due to motivational and cultural backgrounds [22–24].

An individual awareness of beauty is growing among people, both teenagers and adults, across the globe. This is essentially one of the leading causative factors moving ahead the market value. Obviously, a surging multiculturalist attitude, particularly in Western countries, has revised some orthodox beauty norms, thus increasing the demand for non-surgical rhinoplasty implants, such as fillers, for nose plastics. Moreover, the pervasive celebrity culture inflating our real world has a significant appeal on the ideal concept of beauty and its self-consciousness, particularly if alongside public admissions of using these procedures with success.

Finally, it is noteworthy to strengthen the concept that certain rhinoplasty approaches greatly ameliorate one's own psychological consideration, driving one to emotional and social benefits. The rhinoplasty market therefore widely reflects the complex dynamics of expectations from a continuously changing and developing world.

REFERENCES

1. Pandeirada JNS, Fernandes NL, Vasconcelos M. Attractiveness of human faces: norms by sex, sexual orientation, age, relationship stability, and own attractiveness judgements. Front Psychol. 2020 Mar 13;11:419.
2. Coetzee V, Greeff JM, Stephen ID, Perrett DI. Cross-cultural agreement in facial attractiveness preferences: the role of ethnicity and gender. PLoS One. 2014 Jul 2;9(7):e99629.
3. Langlois JH, Kalakanis L, Rubenstein AJ, Larson A, Hallam M, Smoot M. Maxims or myths of beauty? A meta-analytic and theoretical review. Psychol Bull. 2000 May;126(3):390–423.
4. Isik AI, Vessel EA. From visual perception to aesthetic appeal: brain responses to aesthetically appealing natural landscape movies. Front Hum Neurosci. 2021 Jul 21;15:676032.
5. Vessel EA, Isik AI, Belfi AM, Stahl JL, Starr GG. The default-mode network represents aesthetic appeal that generalizes across visual domains. Proc Natl Acad Sci USA. 2019 Sep 17;116(38):19155–19164.
6. Zhao X, Wang J, Li J, Luo G, Li T, Chatterjee A, Zhang W, He X. The neural mechanism of aesthetic judgments of dynamic landscapes: an fMRI study. Sci Rep. 2020 Nov 27;10(1):20774.
7. Leder H, Mitrovic A, Goller J. How beauty determines gaze! Facial attractiveness and gaze duration in images of real world scenes. Iperception. 2016 Aug 23;7(4):2041669516664355.
8. Mitrovic A, Goller J, Tinio PPL, Leder H. How relationship status and sociosexual orientation influence the link between facial attractiveness and visual attention. PLoS One. 2018 Nov 14;13(11):e0207477.
9. Mitrovic A, Tinio PP, Leder H. Consequences of beauty: effects of rater sex and sexual orientation on the visual exploration and evaluation of attractiveness in real world scenes. Front Hum Neurosci. 2016 Mar 21;10:122.
10. Luo Q, Yu M, Li Y, Mo L. The neural correlates of integrated aesthetics between moral and facial beauty. Sci Rep. 2019 Feb 13;9(1):1980.
11. Chatterjee A, Thomas A, Smith SE, Aguirre GK. The neural response to facial attractiveness. Neuropsychology. 2009 Mar;23(2):135–143.
12. Eggerstedt M, Rhee J, Urban MJ, Mangahas A, Smith RM, Revenaugh PC. Beauty is in the eye of the follower: facial aesthetics in the age of social media. Am J Otolaryngol. 2020 Nov–Dec;41(6):102643.
13. Bueller H. Ideal facial relationships and goals. Facial Plast Surg. 2018 Oct;34(5):458–465.
14. Hönn M, Göz G. The ideal of facial beauty: a review. J Orofac Orthop. 2007 Jan;68(1):6–16.
15. Cellerino A. Psychobiology of facial attractiveness. J Endocrinol Invest. 2003;26(3 Suppl):45–48.
16. Kiekens RM, Kuijpers-Jagtman AM, van 't Hof MA, van 't Hof BE, Straatman H, Maltha JC. Facial esthetics in adolescents and its relationship to "ideal" ratios and angles. Am J Orthod Dentofacial Orthop. 2008 Feb;133(2):188.e1–8.
17. Rhodes G. The evolutionary psychology of facial beauty. Annu Rev Psychol. 2006;57:199–226.
18. Naini FB, Moss JP, Gill DS. The enigma of facial beauty: esthetics, proportions, deformity, and controversy. Am J Orthod Dentofacial Orthop. 2006 Sep;130(3):277–282.
19. Baudouin JY, Tiberghien G. Symmetry, averageness, and feature size in the facial attractiveness of women. Acta Psychol (Amst). 2004 Nov;117(3):313–332.
20. Bayat M, Bahrami N, Mesgari H. Rhinoplasty with fillers and fat grafting. Oral Maxillofac Surg Clin North Am. 2021 Feb;33(1):83–110.
21. Balai E, Jolly K, Bhamra N, Osborne MS, Barraclough J. The changing face of rhinology in the NHS: a study of septoplasty, septorhinoplasty and rhinoplasty hospital episode statistics. Ann R Coll Surg Engl. 2021 Apr;103(4):291–295.
22. Alotaibi AS. Demographic and cultural differences in the acceptance and pursuit of cosmetic surgery: a systematic literature review. Plast Reconstr Surg Glob Open. 2021 Mar 24;9(3):e3501.
23. Al Ghadeer HA, Al Alwan MA, Al Amer MA, Alali FJ, Alkhars GA, Alabdrabulrida SA, Al Shabaan HR, Buhlaigah AM, Al Hewishel MA, Alabdrabalnabi HA. Impact of self-esteem and self-perceived body image on the acceptance of cosmetic surgery. Cureus. 2021 Oct 16;13(10):e18825.
24. Marinozzi S, Sanese G, Messineo D, Raposio E, Codolini L, Carbonaro R, Cervelli V. The art of rhinoplasty: researching technical and cultural foundations of Western world rhinosurgery, from the middle ages to the renaissance. Aesthetic Plast Surg. 2021 Dec;45(6):2886–2895.

CHAPTER 1.2

Hyaluronic Acid Fillers

Dario Bertossi, Riccardo Nocini, and Ali Pirayesh

Hyaluronic acid (HA) fillers used in aesthetic indications typically consist of chemically crosslinked HA molecules, resulting in a hydrogel that is less susceptible to enzymatic degradation (i.e., it has a longer duration) and has improved rheologic properties compared with uncrosslinked HA [25,26]. Variations in the manufacturing processes, such as the degree of crosslinking, crosslinking conditions (temperature, pH), molecular weight of the starting HA, and post-crosslinking modifications (sieving/homogenization, addition of lidocaine, etc.), can impact filler characteristics [27–31]. Understanding the range of HA filler products from the standpoint of their rheologic and physicochemical characteristics, can provide an initial framework for predicting treatment outcomes [32] and assist clinicians in selecting the appropriate attributes for each treated facial area [33,34]. Rheologic and physicochemical properties of HA fillers impact performance characteristics (i.e., lift capacity, resistance to deformation, and tissue integration), which, along with injection technique (i.e., injection plane, location, volume) and the interaction of the filler with the surrounding tissues, may affect clinical outcomes [34].

Once injected, HA fillers encounter various forces, such as relative movement (shear) between tissue layers (skin, muscles, fat pads, bone), gravity, and/or compression (by overlying tissues or external pressure) [34]. Therefore, assessing the behavior of fillers in response to mechanical stress provides clinically relevant information [35]. Rheology, the study of the way with which a material deforms and reacts under mechanical stress, allows for this assessment [36]. Four rheologic parameters may be used as the primary measures of a gel's viscoelastic properties: G^* (a measure of the overall viscoelastic properties), G' (a measure of the elastic properties), G'' (a measure of the viscous properties), and $\tan \delta$ (tan delta, a measure of the ratio of the elastic to viscous properties) [36–38].

The previously described rheologic and physicochemical characteristics are important for developing an understanding of HA filler characteristics, allowing selection of fillers that may be suited for each indication and facial area. However, for values to be meaningful for direct comparison, studies of the rheologic and physicochemical properties must be carried out using consistent methodology.

To obtain information on the rheologic and physicochemical properties of HA filler products across manufacturers, different products were tested for G', G'', $\tan \delta$, cohesivity, and water uptake using the standardized methods described by Hee and colleagues [34]. Briefly, fillers were tested using a rheometer at 5 Hz with 0.8% strain; resistance to compression to assess cohesivity was measured using maximum normal force at 0.8 mm/min for 2 minutes, and water uptake was measured by dyeing any buffer that was not taken up by the filler gel and calculating the maximum absorption ratio as the percentage difference between the initial and final gel percentage [34].

For example, in areas of the upper face where filling and volume restoration are required, as in the temporal fossa [39–41], the HA filler should have high elasticity or resistance to deformation (G') and medium to high cohesivity. To address the forehead contour, the filler chosen should have a medium to high G' and a low to medium cohesivity [42], which would allow for molding and some degree of spread upon injection.

In the case of the midface, the infraorbital area is characterized by very thin tissue overlying bone with skin that is only a few millimeters thick. Therefore, a filler for this area should have low to medium elasticity or resistance to deformation (G') and a low cohesivity for ease of spreadability and to prevent overcorrection, lumps, and bumps [43–45]. As the aesthetic visage of the periorbital region is particularly sensitive to slight volume revisions, surgeons should use filler types with low water uptake in order to reduce the risk of puffiness and swelling below the eyes [46–48].

The zygomatic and submalar areas are subject to dynamic contraction forces of the lip and cheek elevators.

Therefore, the fillers used in these areas need to have a medium to high elastic modulus (G′) to resist to shearing and medium to high cohesivity to withstand compression forces of the overlying tissue and to maintain projection [49].

This degree of cohesivity is essential to ensure minimal separation and avoid product displacement that may occur after repetitive contraction of the overlying musculature [50]. In order to give rise to a projection, any filler employed in the midface should be endowed with a high lifting ability. Many HA fillers having previously described physicochemical and rheology hallmarks resulted in effective in the treatment of the midface.

For treating the lower face, the method is quite different. The lower face is characterized by a significant degree of dynamic, with reduction in volume and in the structural support in the region, often resulting in accordion lines, marionette lines, or nasolabial folds. This requires a further consideration of distinct rheologic characteristics, such as medium elasticity (G′) and low to medium cohesivity [51,52], with a moderate lift capacity. The ideal filler for this region would need to be easily moldable, have low projection, be non-palpable, and integrate well with facial movement, as it will be mostly subjected to shearing and mild compression forces. However, to correct severe folds, a filler with higher cohesivity is recommended, although it could be harder to mold after injection.

The lips are treated with HA with medium elasticity. To enhance the lips, fillers are usually described as soft, i.e., having low to medium elasticity (G′) and low to medium cohesivity, since the challenge in this area is to avoid edges and bumps. Also, a low swelling factor is usually recommended to avoid unnatural-looking results [53,54]. For a smoothing effect, lip fillers require lower lift capacity and easy moldability [55,56]. Increasing the cohesivity from low to medium or even to high will contribute to projection and volumization [56]. There are a number of HA fillers with the appropriate combination of elasticity, cohesivity, softness, and water uptake that have been shown to be effective for treating the lips.

Areas such as the jaw, chin, or the nasal dorsum are characterized by a low shear stress, yet with high compression, with tense skin and musculature over bone structures. Thus, the filler of choice to enhance contouring and provide structure should have high elasticity (G′) and medium to high cohesivity and provide high lift capacity and resistance to deformation. A filler with these features should make any lateral spreading minimal, thus maintaining a keen vertical projection over time. Several products showing a proper balance of the many rheologic features resulted in a good efficacy for these skin areas in many clinical trials.

HA fillers are able to ameliorate wrinkles on the face surface via the filling process in shallow lines, with subsequent smoothness of the skin and leading to an outcome appearing as an ameliorated skin quality. Fillers with low HA concentration that exhibit low to medium elasticity (G′) combined with low cohesivity are best suited to treat superficial fine lines, such as those in the periorbital and perioral areas [57–59]. As mentioned earlier, HA fillers with low cohesivity are generally easier to mold and have increased spread in tissues. Because any of these fillers are often injected on surfaces, they need reduced lift capability, low resistance to any deformability, and efficient tissue integrability. This kind of filler may integrate better with the surrounding tissue, they can exhibit good performance alongside a dynamic movement, and they are less likely to result in apparent edges with bumps or palpability.

BIBLIOGRAPHY

25. Kablik J, Monheit GD, Yu L, Chang G, Gershkovich J. Comparative physical properties of hyaluronic acid dermal fillers. Dermatol Surg. 2009 Feb;35 Suppl 1:302–12.
26. Bacos JT, Dayan SH. Superficial dermal fillers with hyaluronic acid. Facial Plast Surg. 2019 Jun;35(3):219–223.
27. Philipp-Dormston WG, Bergfeld D, Sommer BM, Sattler G, Cotofana S, Snozzi P, Wollina U, Hoffmann KPJ, Salavastru C, Fritz K. Consensus statement on prevention and management of adverse effects following rejuvenation procedures with hyaluronic acid-based fillers. J Eur Acad Dermatol Venereol. 2017 Jul;31(7):1088–1095.
28. Faivre J, Gallet M, Tremblais E, Trévidic P, Bourdon F. Advanced concepts in rheology for the evaluation of hyaluronic acid-based soft tissue fillers. Dermatol Surg. 2021 May 1;47(5):e159–e167.
29. Edsman K, Nord LI, Ohrlund A, Lärkner H, Kenne AH. Gel properties of hyaluronic acid dermal fillers. Dermatol Surg. 2012 Jul;38(7 Pt 2):1170–1179.
30. Fagien S, Bertucci V, von Grote E, Mashburn JH. Rheologic and physicochemical properties used to differentiate injectable hyaluronic acid filler products. Plast Reconstr Surg. 2019 Apr;143(4):707e–720e.
31. Sundaram H, Cassuto D. Biophysical characteristics of hyaluronic acid soft-tissue fillers and their relevance to aesthetic applications. Plast Reconstr Surg. 2013 Oct;132(4 Suppl 2):5S–21S.
32. Fagien S, Bertucci V, von Grote E, Mashburn JH. Rheologic and physicochemical properties used to differentiate injectable hyaluronic acid filler products. Plast Reconstr Surg. 2019 Apr;143(4):707e–720e.
33. Kapoor KM, Saputra DI, Porter CE, Colucci L, Stone C, Brenninkmeijer EEA, Sloane J, Sayed K, Winaya KK, Bertossi D. Treating aging changes of facial anatomical layers with hyaluronic acid fillers. Clin Cosmet Investig Dermatol. 2021 Aug 26;14:1105–1118.
34. Michaud T. Rheology of hyaluronic acid and dynamic facial rejuvenation: topographical specificities. J Cosmet Dermatol. 2018 Oct;17(5):736–743.
35. Hee CK, Shumate GT, Narurkar V, Bernardin A, Messina DJ. Rheological properties and in vivo performance characteristics of soft tissue fillers. Dermatol Surg. 2015 Dec;41 Suppl 1:S373–S381.

36. Heitmiller K, Ring C, Saedi N. Rheologic properties of soft tissue fillers and implications for clinical use. J Cosmet Dermatol. 2021 Jan;20(1):28–34.
37. Choi MS. Basic rheology of dermal filler. Arch Plast Surg. 2020 Jul;47(4):301–304.
38. Tezel A, Fredrickson GH. The science of hyaluronic acid dermal fillers. J Cosmet Laser Ther. 2008 Mar;10(1):35–42.
39. Baumann LS, Weisberg EM, Mayans M, Arcuri E. Open label study evaluating efficacy, safety, and effects on perception of age after injectable 20 mg/mL hyaluronic acid gel for volumization of facial temples. J Drugs Dermatol. 2019 Jan 1;18(1):67–74.
40. Wollina U, Goldman A. Correction of tear trough deformity by hyaluronic acid soft tissue filler placement inferior to the lateral orbital thickening. Dermatol Ther. 2021 Sep;34(5):e15045.
41. Hevia O, Cohen BH, Howell DJ. Safety and efficacy of a cohesive polydensified matrix hyaluronic acid for the correction of infraorbital hollow: an observational study with results at 40 weeks. J Drugs Dermatol. 2014 Sep;13(9):1030–1036.
42. Bertossi D, Lanaro L, Dell'Acqua I, Albanese M, Malchiodi L, Nocini PF. Injectable profiloplasty: forehead, nose, lips, and chin filler treatment. J Cosmet Dermatol. 2019 Aug;18(4):976–984.
43. Lorenc ZP, Öhrlund Å, Edsman K. Factors affecting the rheological measurement of hyaluronic acid gel fillers. J Drugs Dermatol. 2017 Sep 1;16(9):876–882.
44. Fallacara A, Manfredini S, Durini E, Vertuani S. Hyaluronic acid fillers in soft tissue regeneration. Facial Plast Surg. 2017 Feb;33(1):87–96. doi: 10.1055/s-0036-1597685. Epub 2017 Feb 22. Erratum in: Facial Plast Surg. 2017 Apr;33(2):244.
45. Ho D, Jagdeo J. Safety and efficacy of a volumizing hyaluronic acid filler for treatment of HIV-associated facial lipoatrophy. JAMA Dermatol. 2017 Jan 1;153(1):61–65.
46. Niforos F, Acquilla R, Ogilvie P, Safa M, Signorini M, Creutz L, Kerson G, Silberberg M. A prospective, open-label study of hyaluronic acid-based filler with lidocaine (VYC-15L) treatment for the correction of infraorbital skin depressions. Dermatol Surg. 2017 Oct;43(10):1271–1280.
47. Sharad J. Dermal fillers for the treatment of tear trough deformity: a review of anatomy, treatment techniques, and their outcomes. J Cutan Aesthet Surg. 2012 Oct;5(4):229–238.
48. Trinh LN, Grond SE, Gupta A. Dermal fillers for tear trough rejuvenation: a systematic review. Facial Plast Surg. 2021 Jun 30. doi: 10.1055/s-0041-1731348.
49. Jones D, Murphy DK. Volumizing hyaluronic acid filler for midface volume deficit: 2-year results from a pivotal single-blind randomized controlled study. Dermatol Surg. 2013 Nov;39(11):1602–1612.
50. Wilson AJ, Taglienti AJ, Chang CS, Low DW, Percec I. Current applications of facial volumization with fillers. Plast Reconstr Surg. 2016 May;137(5):872e–889e.
51. Monheit G, Beer K, Hardas B, Grimes PE, Weichman BM, Lin V, Murphy DK. Safety and effectiveness of the hyaluronic acid dermal filler VYC-17.5L for nasolabial folds: results of a randomized, controlled study. Dermatol Surg. 2018 May;44(5):670–678.
52. Monheit G, Kaufman-Janette J, Joseph JH, Shamban A, Dover JS, Smith S. Efficacy and safety of two resilient hyaluronic acid fillers in the treatment of moderate-to-severe nasolabial folds: a 64-week, prospective, multicenter, controlled, randomized, double-blinded, and within-subject study. Dermatol Surg. 2020 Dec;46(12):1521–1529.
53. Eccleston D, Murphy DK. Juvéderm(®) Volbella™ in the perioral area: a 12-month prospective, multicenter, open-label study. Clin Cosmet Investig Dermatol. 2012;5:167–172.
54. Dayan S, Bruce S, Kilmer S, Dover JS, Downie JB, Taylor SC, Skorupa A, Murphy DK. Safety and effectiveness of the hyaluronic acid filler, HYC-24L, for lip and perioral augmentation. Dermatol Surg. 2015 Dec;41 Suppl 1:S293–301.
55. Fischer TC, Sattler G, Gauglitz GG. Hyaluron filler containing lidocaine on a CPM basis for lip augmentation: reports from practical experience. Facial Plast Surg. 2016 Jun;32(3):283–288.
56. Wende FJ, Gohil S, Nord LI, Helander Kenne A, Sandström C. 1D NMR methods for determination of degree of cross-linking and BDDE substitution positions in HA hydrogels. Carbohydr Polym. 2017 Feb 10;157:1525–1530.
57. Niforos F, Ogilvie P, Cavallini M, Leys C, Chantrey J, Safa M, Abrams S, Hopfinger R, Marx A. VYC-12 injectable gel is safe and effective for improvement of facial skin topography: a prospective study. Clin Cosmet Investig Dermatol. 2019 Oct 24;12:791–798.
58. Black JM, Gross TM, Murcia CL, Jones DH. Cohesive polydensified matrix hyaluronic acid for the treatment of etched-in fine facial lines: a 6-month, open-label clinical trial. Dermatol Surg. 2018 Jul;44(7):1002–1011.
59. Sundaram H, Fagien S. Cohesive polydensified matrix hyaluronic acid for fine lines. Plast Reconstr Surg. 2015 Nov;136(5 Suppl):149S–163S.

CHAPTER **1.3**

Botulinum Toxin

Dario Bertossi, Riccardo Nocini, and Ali Pirayesh

Botulinum toxin (Botox), consisting of a neuromuscular blocking protein produced by the anaerobic bacterium *Clostridium botulinum,* which is adapted to be safely injected into patients, is used in aesthetic medicine to target facial areas such as the forehead, crow's feet, medial eyebrows (corrugator muscle), the jowl, and platysma neckbands [60]. Recent statistics estimated that treatment with botulinum toxin is probably the most performed in aesthetic medicine, only followed by hyaluronic acid (HA) fillers [61,62]. Three different formulations of botulinum toxin with distinct molecular, biochemical, and physiological features have been approved for aesthetic use in Italy. The formulations have different profiles of efficacy and safety, and potency units of each formulation are not interchangeable with other preparations of botulinum toxin [63].

Onabotulinum toxin A was the first formulation of botulinum toxin available worldwide and is now approved by the Food and Drug Administration (FDA) in adult patients for the temporary improvement in the appearance of a) moderate-to-severe glabellar lines associated with corrugator and/or procerus muscle activity, b) moderate-to-severe lateral canthal lines associated with orbicularis oculi activity, and c) moderate-to-severe forehead lines associated with frontalis muscle activity.

In Italy, it is currently licensed for the temporary improvement of glabellar lines and lateral canthal lines in adult patients when there is a significant psychological impact [64]. Both the safety and effectiveness of any approved botulinum toxin have been thoroughly investigated and recently reviewed [65]. The precision of the treatment in terms of patient assessment, identification and number of injection sites, doses, injected volumes, and recommendations to the patient is essential to achieve good aesthetic results and replicate the success. Many consensus guidelines and recommendations and guidelines have been reported in recent years. H. Sundaram et al. recently published two papers including botulinum toxin treatment and complication management and combined treatment with botulinum toxin and fillers, highlighting how to optimize the treatment in different patient populations. The consensus recommendations published by J. Carruthers et al. are also focused on combined treatments and involve not only botulinum toxin and fillers but also energy devices [66]. International guidelines or recommendations could sometimes be difficult to apply in real life due to different standards of beauty, patient needs, and culture. This phenomenon led, over the years, to the publication of different consensus recommendations in several countries [67–69]

BUNNY LINES

Bunny lines are generated predominantly from the paramedial portion of the transverse muscle of the nose, which causes oblique wrinkles in a lateral-medial direction from top to bottom. The dose for the injection site is 2 U per side. The injection is carried out with an inclination of 45 degrees with respect to the cutaneous plane, with the direction from the bottom to the top. For the treatment of bunny lines, we recommend the use of two superficial injection sites in the center of the affected area, with a depth equal to only the tip of the needle. The muscle, in fact, is located immediately below the skin of the nasal wall. It is recommended not to carry out the inoculum in a too lateral position as to not interfere with the function of the elevator of the upper lip and of the nasal wing. Although, the elevator of the upper lip and the nasal wing is associated with the formation of bunny lines; however, treatment is not recommended in order to avoid ptosis of the upper lip. On the contrary, it can be combined with treatment of the procerus muscle, responsible for horizontal wrinkles at the root of the nose (refer to the glabella section for its specific treatment).

SAGGING NASAL TIP

The target muscle for treating a drooping nasal tip is the depressant of the nasal septum. In the presence of hypertonia, the depressor of the nasal septum generates the lowering of the tip of the nose, and this lowering can be further accentuated when smiling. For the drooping nasal tip, we recommend that the treatment be carried out in a single-site injection, with a dose of 2–4 U, in both men and women. The 12-mm, 30-G needle should be inserted halfway through its own length at the base of the columella, with a long orientation with the bisector of the nasolabial angle. Patients undergoing this treatment end up with a pleasing rotation towards the high variable degree of the nasal tip, with enlargement of the nasolabial angle and, above all, the rotation is eliminated of the same downward during talking and smiling. During clinical evaluation, it is necessary to pay attention to patient selection. It is advisable to avoid treatment of the drooping nasal tip in patients with an upper lip that is already excessively long. It is also necessary to verify that the lowered position of the tip has a component muscle and is not, on the other hand, supported exclusively from the nasal septum. In the latter case, the treatment would not lead to any positive outcome.

BIBLIOGRAPHY

60. Mendez-Eastman SK. BOTOX: a review. Plast Surg Nurs. 2003 Summer;23(2):64–69. doi: 10.1097/00006527-200323020-00006.
61. Bertossi D, Cavallini M, Cirillo P, Piero Fundarò S, Quartucci S, Sciuto C, Tonini D, Trocchi G, Signorini M. Italian consensus report on the aesthetic use of onabotulinum toxin A. J Cosmet Dermatol. 2018 Oct;17(5):719–730.
62. The American Society for Aesthetic Plastic Surgery (ASAPS). Cosmetic surgery national data bank. Statistics, 2016. Available at: www.surge ry.org/sites/default/files/ASAPS-Stats2016.pdf. Accessed March 1, 2017.
63. Raspaldo H, Baspeyras M, Bellity P, Dallara JM, Gassia V, Niforos FR, Belhaouari L, Consensus Group. Upper- and mid-face anti-aging treatment and prevention using onabotulinumtoxin A: the 2010 multidisciplinary French consensus—part 1. J Cosmet Dermatol. 2011 Mar;10(1):36–50.
64. Bertossi D, Cavallini M, Cirillo P, Piero Fundarò S, Quartucci S, Sciuto C, Tonini D, Trocchi G, Signorini M. Italian consensus report on the aesthetic use of onabotulinum toxin A. J Cosmet Dermatol. 2018 Oct;17(5):719–730.
65. Cohen JL, Scuderi N. Safety and patient satisfaction of abobotulinumtoxin a for aesthetic use: a systematic review. Aesthet Surg J. 2017 May 1;37(suppl_1):S32–S44.
66. Carruthers J, Burgess C, Day D, Fabi SG, Goldie K, Kerscher M, Nikolis A, Pavicic T, Rho NK, Rzany B, Sattler G, Sattler S, Seo K, Werschler WP, Carruthers A. Consensus recommendations for combined aesthetic interventions in the face using botulinum toxin, fillers, and energy-based devices. Dermatol Surg. 2016 May;42(5):586–597.
67. Kane M, Donofrio L, Ascher B, Hexsel D, Monheit G, Rzany B, Weiss R. Expanding the use of neurotoxins in facial aesthetics: a consensus panel's assessment and recommendations. J Drugs Dermatol. 2010 Jan;9(1 Suppl):s7–22.
68. Raspaldo H, Baspeyras M, Bellity P, Dallara JM, Gassia V, Niforos FR, Belhaouari L, Consensus Group. Upper- and mid-face anti-aging treatment and prevention using onabotulinumtoxin A: the 2010 multidisciplinary French consensus—part 1. J Cosmet Dermatol. 2011 Mar;10(1):36–50.
69. Raspaldo H, Niforos FR, Gassia V, Dallara JM, Bellity P, Baspeyras M, Belhaouari L, Consensus Group. Lower-face and neck antiaging treatment and prevention using onabotulinumtoxin A: the 2010 multidisciplinary French consensus—part 2. J Cosmet Dermatol. 2011 Jun;10(2):131–149.

CHAPTER 1.4

Combined Devices

Dario Bertossi and Salvatore Chirumbolo

Aesthetic medicine and non-surgical rhinoplasty can often rely also on combined approaches and devices, which may include, besides hyaluronic acid (HA) fillers and BoNTa (botulinum toxin), physical techniques adapted to achieve the best aesthetic and rejuvenation outcome [70]. Merging different aesthetic interventions together in an expert combination of refining techniques is a widespread habit in the clinical practice dealing with non-surgical rhinoplasty and aesthetics, despite the controversial consideration that optimal results coming from this approach are rarely reported in the medical literature and at scientific meetings due to the difficulty in standardizing and performing the study. The majority of studies to date, which are addressed in the use of combined aesthetic interventions, are based on Caucasian models of the human population, whereas individuals coming from different ethnicities vary in both baseline facial anatomy and facial appearance, generating fundamental issues to be considered when a combined aesthetic practice is planned [71–73].

To achieve the optimal outcome, the selection of the most appropriate techniques and devices is of utmost importance, along with the physician's expertise, which should ensure their correct use. Several consensus conferences were planned to recommend the optimal combination of different techniques—at least two of them for assessing the ideal sequence of botulinum, HA filler, calcium hydroxyapatite, and energy-based devices [74–77].

The use of lasers can be refined to target the defined type of tissues and different cutaneous depths on the basis of various scattering and absorption profiles of the tissue of interest [78]. In this perspective, any desired aesthetic effect depends on the tissue ability and degree of light energy absorbance, in addition to the expert skill of the surgeon, considering also that endogenous chromogens (hemoglobin, melanin, and water itself with dissolved proteins) determine the various levels of wavelength absorbance and reflection, a pattern to be crucially considered in a combined aesthetic approach. For example, in the case of sun damage, skin tightening, burns, and deep rhytids a CO_2 laser (10,000 nm) is recommended; for deep hemangiomas an Nd:YAG laser (1064 nm, 1320 nm, or 1540 nm) is recommended; and for acne, vascular lesions, and rosacea an intense pulsed light laser (400–1200 nm) is suggested [78].

The role of HA in combined devices for aesthetic medicine is characterized by its ability to gather water molecules. For example, the VYCROSS technology, from Allergan Inc., gives HA fillers much more efficacious crosslinking, thus affecting the rheology of the product and its hydrophilic properties [79]. HA fillers therefore present a significant amount of light absorption from wavelengths higher than 1000 nm, since for HA the molar extinction coefficient increases linearly with increasing wavelength. Moreover, for lasers and intense light devices, the reference system lies on the different times of emission, which can be measured from picoseconds (ps) to seconds (s), where the longer the light pulse, the higher the penetration range into tissues [78]. Recent reports reviewed the practice of combined pulsed light and laser devices with HA fillers [79–83].

The number of publications on the use of sonography in dermatology and aesthetic medicine has grown recently [84]. Their authors pointed to the usefulness of both classic scanners equipped with linear transducers and high-frequency scanners with mechanical transducers [84,85]. Ultrasonography with Doppler options creates new diagnostic possibilities in evaluating both healthy and pathological skin [86,87]. A large number of modalities can be used for the evaluation of microcirculation in the skin, such as Color Power Angio (CPA), color Doppler (CD), microflow imaging (MFI), and pulsed wave Doppler (PWD). Interestingly, MFI is available only in scanners endowed with high-class standard ultrasound devices.

BIBLIOGRAPHY

70. Fabi S, Pavicic T, Braz A, Green JB, Seo K, van Loghem JA. Combined aesthetic interventions for prevention of facial ageing, and restoration and beautification of face and body. Clin Cosmet Investig Dermatol. 2017 Oct 30;10:423–429.
71. Rho NK, Chang YY, Chao YY, Furuyama N, Huang PYC, Kerscher M, Kim HJ, Park JY, Peng HLP, Rummaneethorn P, Rzany B, Sundaram H, Wong CH, Yang Y, Prasetyo AD. Consensus recommendations for optimal augmentation of the Asian face with hyaluronic acid and calcium hydroxylapatite fillers. Plast Reconstr Surg. 2015 Nov;136(5):940–956.
72. Sundaram H, Huang PH, Hsu NJ, Huh CH, Wu WT, Wu Y, Cassuto D, Kerscher MJ, Seo KK, Pan-Asian Aesthetics Toxin Consensus Group. Aesthetic applications of botulinum toxin a in Asians: an international, multidisciplinary, pan-Asian consensus. Plast Reconstr Surg Glob Open. 2016 Dec 7;4(12):e872.
73. Brissett AE, Naylor MC. The aging African-American face. Facial Plast Surg. 2010 May;26(2):154–163.
74. Carruthers J, Burgess C, Day D, Fabi SG, Goldie K, Kerscher M, Nikolis A, Pavicic T, Rho NK, Rzany B, Sattler G, Sattler S, Seo K, Werschler WP, Carruthers A. Consensus recommendations for combined aesthetic interventions in the face using botulinum toxin, fillers, and energy-based devices.
75. Fabi SG, Burgess C, Carruthers A, Carruthers J, Day D, Goldie K, Kerscher M, Nikolis A, Pavicic T, Rho NK, Rzany B, Sattler S, Seo K, Werschler WP, Sattler G. Consensus recommendations for combined aesthetic interventions using botulinum toxin, fillers, and microfocused ultrasound in the neck, décolletage, hands, and other areas of the body. Dermatol Surg. 2016 Oct;42(10):1199–1208.
76. de Almeida AT, Figueredo V, da Cunha ALG, Casabona G, Costa de Faria JR, Alves EV, Sato M, Branco A, Guarnieri C, Palermo E. Consensus recommendations for the use of hyperdiluted calcium hydroxyapatite (radiesse) as a face and body biostimulatory agent. Plast Reconstr Surg Glob Open. 2019 Mar 14;7(3):e2160.
77. Chao YYY, Chhabra C, Corduff N, Fabi SG, Kerscher M, Lam SCK, Pavicic T, Rzany B, Peng PHL, Suwanchinda A, Tseng FW, Seo KK. Pan-Asian consensus-key recommendations for adapting the world congress of dermatology consensus on combination treatment with injectable fillers, toxins, and ultrasound devices in Asian patients. J Clin Aesthet Dermatol. 2017 Aug;10(8):16–27.
78. Urdiales-Gálvez F, Martín-Sánchez S, Maíz-Jiménez M, Castellano-Miralla A, Lionetti-Leone L. Concomitant use of hyaluronic acid and laser in facial rejuvenation. Aesthetic Plast Surg. 2019 Aug;43(4):1061–1070.
79. Philipp-Dormston WG, Hilton S, Nathan M. A prospective, open-label, multicenter, observational, postmarket study of the use of a 15 mg/mL hyaluronic acid dermal filler in the lips. J Cosmet Dermatol. 2014 Jun;13(2):125–134.
80. Cuerda-Galindo E, Palomar-Gallego MA, Linares-Garcíavaldecasas R. Are combined same-day treatments the future for photorejuvenation? Review of the literature on combined treatments with lasers, intense pulsed light, radiofrequency, botulinum toxin, and fillers for rejuvenation. J Cosmet Laser Ther. 2015 Feb;17(1):49–54.
81. Langelier N, Beleznay K, Woodward J. Rejuvenation of the upper face and periocular region: combining neuromodulator, facial filler, laser, light, and energy-based therapies for optimal results. Dermatol Surg. 2016 May;42 Suppl 2:S77–S82.
82. Vanaman M, Fabi SG, Cox SE. Neck rejuvenation using a combination approach: our experience and a review of the literature. Dermatol Surg. 2016 May;42 Suppl 2:S94–S100.
83. Chan CS, Saedi N, Mickle C, Dover JS. Combined treatment for facial rejuvenation using an optimized pulsed light source followed by a fractional non-ablative laser. Lasers Surg Med. 2013 Sep;45(7):405–409.
84. Polańska A, Dańczak-Pazdrowska A, Jałowska M, Żaba R, Adamski Z. Current applications of high-frequency ultrasonography in dermatology. Postepy Dermatol Alergol. 2017 Dec;34(6):535–542.
85. Polańska A, Dańczak-Pazdrowska A, Jałowska M, Żaba R, Adamski Z. Current applications of high-frequency ultrasonography in dermatology. Postepy Dermatol Alergol. 2017 Dec;34(6):535–542.
86. Scotto di Santolo M, Sagnelli M, Mancini M, Scalvenzi M, Delfino M, Schonauer F, Molea G, Ayala F, Salvatore M. High-resolution color-Doppler ultrasound for the study of skin growths. Arch Dermatol Res. 2015 Sep;307(7):559–566.
87. Barcaui Ede O, Carvalho AC, Lopes FP, Piñeiro-Maceira J, Barcaui CB. High frequency ultrasound with color Doppler in dermatology. An Bras Dermatol. 2016 May–Jun;91(3):262–273.

CHAPTER **1.5**

The HA Filler Market

Dario Bertossi, Riccardo Nocini, and Ali Pirayesh

Injections of hyaluronic acid (HA) filler for soft tissue augmentation and facial rejuvenation can be considered the second most common non-surgical aesthetic practice since 2019, accounting for about 4.3 million clinical procedures worldwide, reaching a 16% increase over the previous year [88]. HA, known also as hyaluronan in its saline form, is a disaccharide polymer composed of D-glucuronic acid and N-acetyl-D-glucosamine, which is commercially used as a filler in several medical aesthetic practices at various formulations [89–95]. The extreme biocompatibility and biodegradability are outstanding hallmarks of any HA filler's success, in addition to its overall biotolerability, safety, affordability, administration capability, hydrophilic features and negligible incidence of possible side effects [96–100].

Any HA filler employed in aesthetic medicine is typically made of biochemically crosslinked hyaluronan molecules, often resulting in a kind of hydrogel, which may prevent further enzymatic degradation, leading to a longer duration and endowed with an improved rheologic property when compared with uncrosslinked HA [101,102]. Various formulas do exist in the HA manufacturing processes, for example, the different degrees of crosslinking, the physical-chemical conditions with which crosslinking is performed (pH, temperature, viscosity, etc.), the molecular weight of the starting hyaluronan, and even any post-crosslinking chemical or physical modifications, such as homogenization or sieving, lidocaine adjunct, and so forth, could have a major impact on HA filler features [103–107].

Any physicochemical and rheological property of HA fillers may affect their performance hallmarks, including tissue targeting and integration, lift capability, resistance, and deformability, which alongside different techniques of injection and the same nature of fillers, should affect any outcome in the clinical setting [108]. As any HA filler is a viscoelastic material, when injected, it encounters many forces, which represent fundamental parameters to assess the overall quality of an HA filler. In this circumstance in order to evaluate and measure the viscoelastic properties of the HA gel formula, some indicators such as G^*, which measures the overall viscoelastic characteristics; G', which evaluates elasticity; G'', which measures the viscosity; and δ, indicating the elastic to viscous ratio are widely employed in HA filler marketing [109–111].

The market of HA has been valued at 8.5 billion USD in 2020 and is forecasted to reach a compound annual growth rate (CAGR) of 7.19% by 2028, starting in 2021. The market size value for 2021 was over 8.87 billion USD, and its revenue forecast for 2028 is estimated at 14.42 billion USD. At a global overview, the United States has the leading role in the revenue sharing, accounting for more than 43% in 2020, expanding at a steady CAGR in the next seven years, thus maintaining its pole position; the increasing demand for minimally invasive aesthetic approaches in plastic surgery alone has to be considered a fundamental engine in this growing rate in the United States. Great expectations are foreseen for the Asia Pacific region, particularly for China, Taiwan, South Korea, and Japan, which are forecast to be the newly increasing markets for HA.

In Europe, the HA fillers market is expected to grow at a CAGR of 6.7% in the period 2021 to 2026, then reaching 1,466.81 million USD in 2026 starting from a rate of 1,060.60 million USD in 2021. This very rapid trend can be caused by a rapid increase in aging in the European population, thus enhancing the volume of demand for facelifts and rejuvenation implants [112,113]. People 80 years or older in the European Community (European Union [EU]) are forecasted to increase from 5.9% to 14.6% from 2020 to 2100.

In a general way, the concept of a "filler" has to be considered an umbrella term, commonly referred to as face fillers, including gel-like chemical substances, usually represented by HA, which are injected beneath specific areas of the facial skin. There are several manufacturers combining different physicochemical properties in HA fillers, for example, increasing crosslinking to enhance elasticity (thus elevating G′) or reducing the distance between different crosslinks in order to obtain a softer or less elastic HA filler (decreasing G′). Otherwise, producers using the same technology and a similar degree of crosslinking may obtain a firmer HA filler simply by increasing the hyaluronan concentration [114].

The market of HA fillers is particularly crowded in terms of novelties and specialties, even for small aesthetic requests. Costs vary from country to country; for example, a lip filler ranges from 550 to 2,000 USD per treatment, a cheek filler from 600 to 1,200 USD, a chin filler from 750 to 1,500 USD, a jawline filler around 3,000 USD, and an undereye filler 1,200 USD [92,93,95,115].

Although these data are questionable, pending the market values, they would give a general idea of the expense related to the different non-surgical face aesthetics approaches at the minimal level of expenditures.

The use of fillers in rhinoplasty in the EU represents a significant proportion (23.7%) of a market size value (global filler market), which in 2020 was worth over 1.09 billion USD, and its forecast for 2026 is 1.4 billion USD [116–118]. HA fillers in rhinoplasty have an overall adverse events (AE) rate of 7.6% on a global survey of 2,488 procedures, with only 0.20% (5 cases) considered severe (ischemic reactions and necrosis) [119]. Furthermore, the major request in non-surgical rhinoplasty is a dorsal hump (44%) [120]. In this perspective, safety assessments are crucial in the HA fillers for rhinoplasty.

Despite the consideration that any underreporting of negligible or minor events should not be ruled out, the three years of post-marketing survey and experience on HA fillers for non-surgical rhinoplasty is able to speak to the safety of these products [121].

Finally, the different rheologic, mechanical, and physicochemical properties of HA fillers have major implications in the different performances resulting in clinics. HA fillers are expected to be stable, feel natural, and fit the different needs of facial areas where applied. For example, HA fillers should have high resistance to deforming stress and high elasticity in the upper face, while in the regions indicated for filling and volume restoration, the infraorbital area should require HA fillers of low to medium elasticity, whereas a medium to high elasticity is required for the zygomatic and submalar areas [122].

Fundamentally, the human face is a highly complex and dynamic structure, a circumstance to be considered when choosing an HA filler. An alignment of different rheological and physicochemical features in different HA fillers should help clinicians and surgeons gain the best performance in terms of outcomes and customer and/or patient satisfaction.

CHAPTER **1.6**

The Botulinum Toxin Market

Dario Bertossi, Riccardo Nocini, and Ali Pirayesh

Recent statistics estimated that treatment with botulinum toxin is probably the most performed in aesthetic medicine, only followed by hyaluronic acid (HA) fillers [124,125].

An increasing demand for enhancing one's own aesthetic appearance has triggered the demand for botulinum injections around the world. The several concerns that people feel about their looks, due to the globalized concept of how to appear healthy, young and appealing made botulinum use rapidly increase in both developed countries and developing ones. Among 2,630,832 non-surgical, minimally invasive cosmetic procedures in the United States, botulinum is on the top of the list with 1,301,823 Botox treatments. The Botox market amounts to 5.5 billion USD, with a forecast expanding a compound annual growth rate (CAGR) of 6.9% (2021–2031) and a trend to 10.7 billion USD in 2031; furthermore, type A botulinum represents at least 99% of the botulinum market worldwide, and its sale accounts for 3% of the total cosmetics expenditures. Notably, the botulinum market has gained an amazing CAGR of 8.2% from 2016 to 2020.

The increase in life expectancy has moved the awareness that cosmetic medicine can actually help people in regaining their youthful appearance, and worldwide the population of elderly people is growing, a circumstance that is enhancing the market demand for botulinum. Moreover, scientific research in the botulinum application is growing. The US National Clinical Trial registry reported more than 312 planned and ongoing randomized controlled trials (RCTs) in botulinum research as of June 18, 2021. Furthermore, in March 2021 a trademark of botulinum products announced that a novel formulation of botulinum, i.e., the Daxibotulinumtoxin A for injection (DAXI), is nearing Food and Drug Administration (FDA) approval [126]. DAXI is a novel type A botulinum toxin (BoNTA), which contains a highly purified 150-kDa core neurotoxin with the peptide RTP004 in place of serum albumin, thus enabling the product with greater stability, longer-lasting effects and reduced side effects [127–129].

In the European Union (EU), the botulinum market has been valued at 4.9 billion USD in 2020; a forecast projection is expecting the botulinum market to reach 9,360.2 million USD by 2029, this increasing by a CAGR of 7.56% (2021–2029). The BoNTA segment may be the major contributor to this positive trend, with 3,393.8 million USD in 2020 and a trend to 6,480 million USD in 2029 (CAGR = 7.56%), whereas the botulinum toxin B segment may reach 2,880.2 million USD but at a slightly higher CAGR (7.58%).

The use of botulinum needs to be well documented by photographic data [124]. In the case of glabellar lines, usually onabotulinum toxin A (BoNTa) targets the corrugator and procerus muscles. Here, the suggested dosage of onabotulinum toxin A is usually 4 units (U) for the medial tops of the corrugator supercilia muscle and for the procerus, whereas 2–4 U are used for the lateral sides of the corrugator supercilii muscle, adopting a whole dose of 12–20 U for female subjects, a dosage that might increase to 25 U (male) and 30 U (female) if a strong muscle mass is present [124]. Moreover, for crow's feet, the recommended total dose of BoNTa should be 12–24 U for women and 18–36 U for men. In the case of crow's feet extending quite far laterally, or when the orbicularis muscle is particularly endowed with strength, 1–2 U are suggested to be injected in two additional bi-sided areas, placed laterally to the previous three sites, reaching a total of up to 44 U in males and 32 U in females [124]. International guidelines or recommendations could be sometimes difficult to apply in real life due to different standards of beauty, patient needs and culture. This phenomenon has led over the years to the publication of different consensus recommendations in several countries [125–132].

CHAPTER 1.7

The Impact of Social Networks

Dario Bertossi, Riccardo Nocini, and Ali Pirayesh

The purpose of a social media presence for any given physician, of course, varies widely—just as it does for anyone curating a platform online. Some may seek to establish themselves as educators on YouTube, while others set out to create a comedy channel on TikTok, or many may be in their office by day while trendsetting as influencers on Instagram by night. In this age of unprecedented communication, in which an accessory appendage like a smart phone is more an essential than a luxury, the rising constant is connection and, in conjunction with this connection, an audience grows; for those who take the Hippocratic Oath in an increasingly complicated world that seemingly demands a social media presence, we argue that there are new spins on old ethical dilemmas.

With the ubiquity of connectivity in mind, the pivotal questions for physicians marketing their skills, personality, and/or product online are: Who are we connecting with? Why are we connecting with them? What are the consequences of connecting with them? Here, we hope to explore some of the potential answers to these questions based on the current literature, remind colleagues of the rapidly evolving ethical responsibilities, and propose future potential areas of research on this topic.

So, for starters, who is currently most often targeted and reached by our digital content? There are observable and measurable changes in the trends of age and gender for those seeking cosmetic consultation. Young adults, here defined as those between 18 and 25 years of age, make up an increasingly large number of patients, especially since 2008 [133].

Additionally, there has been a slow but statistically significant increase in men of this age group seeking hyaluronic acid (HA) fillers and botulinum injections [134] over this same time frame. Although these findings are likely intuitive, there is now a concretely demonstrated shift in the field.

From a social media perspective in this industry, this means that professionals and patients alike are seeing more of the faces from this demographic going viral. This demographic, while more health-literate than previous generations, also consume social media at a higher rate and for different reasons—interestingly, they are being found to overlap online sites and apps with health education [135].

This neatly fits into one of the primary "whys" of using social media in facial cosmetics, which is education and demonstration. Entering search terms such as "botox", "filler injections", or "liquid rhinoplasty" on online search engines generates more ads, med-spa addresses, and viral media clips than articles about indications, procedures, and complications. However, this is not the case on all platforms and has allowed for alternative media to fill the void created by the lack of written informational material; searching "botox treatment" on YouTube, for instance, populates almost exclusively educational material for the first dozen videos. These uploads include tutorials, demonstrations, and background on any specific cosmetic procedure that can be searched, with all content, including sources for the creators, layering the business perspective back into the expository.

Additionally, these alternative online platforms are the fastest-growing and most accessible medium for the largest demographic seeking procedures. Though taking different shapes across a huge spectrum, using social media to promote a medical practice is almost a necessity; considering that younger professionals are more likely to use social media and the most likely to seek new patients, this is a logical marriage. Social media platforms are also optimal marketing platforms, as cosmetic interventions rely heavily on pictures to demonstrate efficacy. Thus, content posted to social media sites made to appear in conjunction with researching a provider on a search engine serves as evidence of skill and positive outcomes.

In short, this leads to a footprint across digital platforms that is akin to authority when deployed astutely. Curated content alone may function as a representation of a physician's credentials that is even more resonant to a prospective patient than a curriculum vitae (CV) and long list of credentials would be. Publishing such content on social media can therefore generate patient volume, given the correlation between patient interest in cosmetic consultations and its rising frequency on social media. That said, it is also widely demonstrated that increased procedural volume drives improved patient outcomes; this is conventionally thought to be explained by increasing operator skill, which decreases complications and improves satisfaction.

Plainly stated, practitioners are subject to the same idle wishes for fame as everyone with access to a camera. More innocently, this may be viewed as the desire to appear accessible and personable, with photos of vacations, meals, and family peppered into reels of Botox and fillers. The extreme of this motivation is more often seen, though, as shameless self-promotion and a lack of self-censorship as building an image of glamor to the point where fiction takes priority over content rounded out by reality. This type of focus on marketing through embellishment also might lead to uploading images processed by photo-editing software. Although there is no current research or data on practitioner-driven uploads of edits before and after, there is an abundant library of available images which even cursorily do not pass as unedited.

This finally leads into our asking and addressing: What are the consequences of an increasing reach via social media? We always hope our colleagues are motivated similarly; we want them to be motivated by a desire to help, heal, and improve people when they seek us out. That said, it is important to never forget that anyone can post anything on the Internet, that not all content is created equal.

There is little, if any, official guidance by professional dermatology bodies on what is appropriate for online platforms in terms of promotion. Plastic surgery governing bodies, for instance, demand a degree of honesty in advertising, prohibiting "before and after photographs that use different lighting, poses or photographic techniques to misrepresent results" and "exaggerated claims intended to create false or unjustified expectations of favorable surgical results" [6].

Obviously, the tech-savvy masses with a degree of celebrity, or even those simply seeking it, are not obliged to follow any such recommendations or restrictions. Photos in which beauty standards and selfies are enhanced by the normalization of filters—such interactions between technology, the untrained eye, and increasing rates of body dysmorphia—are contributing to a culture of cosmetic-seeking behavior. On one hand, this fosters a culture of acceptance; we have been presented with, in some cases, an opportunity for early intervention in young adults who now see cosmetic procedures as healthy and normal. In fact, some research suggests that younger people prefer that their cosmetic interventions be noticeable. Given the pro-social nature of promoting beauty, wellness, and confidence, this can naturally be the case when we seek to enhance a person's best baseline attributes.

On the other hand, this untested culture leads to an attitude of desensitization towards unnatural, abnormal beauty standards becoming the new normal. This allows for those practitioners primarily seeking profit, as opposed to the betterment of patients, to prey upon those with an aesthetic addiction at an earlier age. In the future, one can easily imagine this leading to a growing number of patients with pillow-facies. In this time when figures like Kylie Jenner claim to have achieved an appearance solely through the lipstick they happen to brand, we must simply say "no" to patients seeking to look specifically like any named icons.

Best practice dictates that we strive to optimize a person's natural beauty—to make them the best version of themselves—not sculpt them into someone else. In this way, we maintain our status as stewards of ethical beauty, keeping the pro-social from being turned into the antisocial. Having a conversation addressing unrealistic expectations is not only ethical but improves both patient and practitioner satisfaction. Content on social media and in-person consultations should discuss the balance between what is feasible, treatment versus excessive treatment, and the need for agreement between patient and practitioner on both points before treatment.

What should occur when it is clear a patient is seeking cosmetic consultation due to body dysmorphia? These patients may benefit aesthetically from procedures, but whether to provide such treatments when the impetus is pathologic is an increasingly pervasive ethical dilemma. Though not a cause of body dysmorphia, social media has been demonstrated to exacerbate it [10]. Flatly, there is no amount of informed consent, no length or detail of conversation, which can ethically or morally justify initiating treatment in patients with this pathology.

This all assumes that moral pitfalls aside, professionals administering cosmetic care are of equal quality and quantity in training. Broad searches on social media for the most common non-surgical facial treatments returns content that is unlikely to clearly state the credentials of a depicted professional as a dermatologist, plastic surgeon, nurse practitioner, or aesthetician. But there is a body of data that in tandem with the substantial growth in a population seeking out non-surgical cosmetic treatments is a proportional gain in the number of untrained, unsupervised practitioners. Inexperienced operators can be found performing in office settings too, but the highest rates of non-physicians administering treatments occur at med-spas.

Although complications are not recorded at increasing rates as of yet, the data clearly purports those complications are more common with treatment from non-physicians—non-physicians, as mentioned, are more likely to be practicing at med-spas than offices and are more likely to be unsupervised in the spa setting. Burns and discoloration from lasers and injections are the most common complications seen in patients post-treatment, pursuing in-office consultation after med-spas; a lack of understanding of either anatomy or manual technique was cited as the most common sources of these complications.

BIBLIOGRAPHY

88. International Society of Aesthetic Plastic Surgery. ISAPS international survey on aesthetic/cosmetic procedures performed in 2019, 2020. Available at: www.isaps.org/wp-content/uploads/2020/12/Global-Survey-2019.pdf. Accessed October 14, 2021.
89. Bukhari SNA, Roswandi NL, Waqas M, Habib H, Hussain F, Khan S, Sohail M, Ramli NA, Thu HE, Hussain Z. Hyaluronic acid, a promising skin rejuvenating biomedicine: a review of recent updates and pre-clinical and clinical investigations on cosmetic and nutricosmetic effects. Int J Biol Macromol. 2018 Dec;120(Pt B):1682–1695.
90. Gutowski KA. Hyaluronic acid fillers: science and clinical uses. Clin Plast Surg. 2016 Jul;43(3):489–496.
91. Moradi A, Watson J. Current concepts in filler injection. Facial Plast Surg Clin North Am. 2015 Nov;23(4):489–494.
92. Cassuto D, Bellia G, Schiraldi C. An overview of soft tissue fillers for cosmetic dermatology: from filling to regenerative medicine. Clin Cosmet Investig Dermatol. 2021 Dec 22;14:1857–1866.
93. Galadari H, Weinkle SH. Injection techniques for midface volumization using soft tissue hyaluronic acid fillers designed for dynamic facial movement. J Cosmet Dermatol. 2021 Dec 28. doi: 10.1111/jocd.14700.
94. Cohen JL, Hicks J, Nogueira A, Lane V, Andriopoulos B. Postmarket safety surveillance of delayed complications for recent FDA-approved hyaluronic acid dermal fillers. Dermatol Surg. 2021 Dec 20. doi: 10.1097/DSS.0000000000003350.
95. Basta SL. Cosmetic fillers: perspectives on the industry. Facial Plast Surg Clin North Am. 2015 Nov;23(4):417–421.
96. Humphrey S, Carruthers J, Carruthers A. Clinical experience with 11,460 mL of a 20-mg/mL, smooth, highly cohesive, viscous hyaluronic acid filler. Dermatol Surg. 2015;41(9):1060–1067.
97. Philipp-Dormston WG, Bergfeld D, Sommer BM, et al. Consensus statement on prevention and management of adverse effects following rejuvenation procedures with hyaluronic acid based fillers. J Eur Acad Dermatol Venereol. 2017;31(7):1088–1095.
98. Snozzi P, van Loghem JAJ. Complication management following rejuvenation procedures with hyaluronic acid fillers-an algorithm-based approach. Plast Reconstr Surg Glob Open. 2018;6(12):e2061.
99. Matarasso SL. Understanding and using hyaluronic acid. Aesthet Surg J. 2004;24(4):361–364.
100. Salwowska NM, Bebenek KA, Żądło DA, Wcisło-Dziadecka DL. Physiochemical properties and application of hyaluronic acid: a systematic review. J Cosmet Dermatol. 2016;15(4):520–526.
101. Kablik J, Monheit GD, Yu L, Chang G, Gershkovich J. Comparative physical properties of hyaluronic acid dermal fillers. Dermatol Surg. 2009;35 Suppl 1:302–312.
102. Bacos JT, Dayan SH. Superficial dermal fillers with hyaluronic acid. Facial Plast Surg. 2019;35(3):219–223.
103. Philipp-Dormston WG, Bergfeld D, Sommer BM, et al. Consensus statement on prevention and management of adverse effects following rejuvenation procedures with hyaluronic acid based fillers. J Eur Acad Dermatol Venereol. 2017;31(7):1088–1095.
104. Faivre J, Gallet M, Tremblais E, Trévidic P, Bourdon F. Advanced concepts in rheology for the evaluation of hyaluronic acid-based soft tissue fillers. Dermatol Surg. 2021;47(5):e159–e167.
105. Edsman K, Nord LI, Ohrlund A, Larkner H, Kenne AH. Gel properties of hyaluronic acid dermal fillers. Dermatol Surg. 2012;38(7 Pt 2):1170–1179.
106. Fagien S, Bertucci V, von Grote E, Mashburn JH. Rheologic and physicochemical properties used to differentiate injectable hyaluronic acid filler products. Plast Reconstr Surg. 2019;143(4):707e–720e.
107. Sundaram H, Cassuto D. Biophysical characteristics of hyaluronic acid soft-tissue fillers and their relevance to aesthetic applications. Plast Reconstr Surg. 2013;132(4 Suppl 2):5S–21S.
108. Michaud T. Rheology of hyaluronic acid and dynamic facial rejuvenation: topographical specificities. J Cosmet Dermatol. 2018;17(5):736–743.
109. Pierre S, Liew S, Bernardin A. Basics of dermal filler rheology. Dermatol Surg. 2015;41(suppl 1):S120–S126.
110. Goldman MP, Few J, Binauld S, Nuñez I, Hee CK, Bernardin A. Evaluation of physicochemical properties following syringe-to-syringe mixing of hyaluronic acid dermal fillers. Dermatol Surg. 2020;46(12):1606–1612.
111. Lorenc ZP, Ohrlund A, Edsman K. Factors affecting the rheological measurement of hyaluronic acid gel fillers. J Drugs Dermatol. 2017;16(9):876–882.
112. Marois G, Bélanger A, Lutz W. Population aging, migration, and productivity in Europe. Proc Natl Acad Sci U S A. 2020 Apr 7;117(14):7690–7695.
113. Bray D, Hopkins C, Roberts DN. A review of dermal fillers in facial plastic surgery. Curr Opin Otolaryngol Head Neck Surg. 2010 Aug;18(4):295–302.
114. Lundgren B, Sandkvist U, Bordier N, Gauthier B. Using a new photo scale to compare product integration of different hyaluronan-based fillers after injection in human ex vivo skin. J Drugs Dermatol. 2018;17(9):982–986.
115. Marois G, Bélanger A, Lutz W. Population aging, migration, and productivity in Europe. Proc Natl Acad Sci U S A. 2020 Apr 7;117(14):7690–7695.
116. Hedén P. Nasal reshaping with hyaluronic acid: an alternative or complement to surgery. Plast Reconstr Surg Glob Open. 2016 Nov 28;4(11):e1120.
117. Bayat M, Bahrami N, Mesgari H. Rhinoplasty with fillers and fat grafting. Oral Maxillofac Surg Clin North Am. 2021 Feb;33(1):83–110.
118. Hopkins ZH, Moreno C, Secrest AM. Influence of social media on cosmetic procedure interest. J Clin Aesthet Dermatol. 2020 Jan;13(1):28–31.

119. Rivkin A. Nonsurgical rhinoplasty using injectable fillers: a safety review of 2488 procedures. Facial Plast Surg Aesthet Med. 2021 Jan–Feb;23(1):6–11.
120. Harb A, Brewster CT. The nonsurgical rhinoplasty: a retrospective review of 5000 treatments. Plast Reconstr Surg. 2020 Mar;145(3):661–667.
121. Cassuto D, Delledonne M, Zaccaria G, Illiano I, Giori AM, Bellia G. Safety assessment of high- and low-molecular-weight hyaluronans (Profhilo®) as derived from worldwide postmarketing data. Biomed Res Int. 2020 Jun 20;2020:8159047.
122. Bertossi D, Lanaro L, Dell'Acqua I, Albanese M, Malchiodi L, Nocini PF. Injectable profiloplasty: forehead, nose, lips, and chin filler treatment. J Cosmet Dermatol. 2019;18(4):976–984.
123. Mendez-Eastman SK. BOTOX: a review. Plast Surg Nurs. 2003 Summer;23(2):64–69. doi: 10.1097/00006527-200323020-00006.
124. Bertossi D, Cavallini M, Cirillo P, Piero Fundarò S, Quartucci S, Sciuto C, Tonini D, Trocchi G, Signorini M. Italian consensus report on the aesthetic use of onabotulinum toxin A. J Cosmet Dermatol. 2018 Oct;17(5):719–730.
125. The American Society for Aesthetic Plastic Surgery (ASAPS). Cosmetic surgery national data bank. Statistics, 2016. Available at: www.surge ry.org/sites/default/files/ASAPS-Stats2016.pdf. Accessed March 1, 2017.
126. Raspaldo H, Baspeyras M, Bellity P, Dallara JM, Gassia V, Niforos FR, Belhaouari L, Consensus Group. Upper- and mid-face anti-aging treatment and prevention using onabotulinumtoxin A: the 2010 multidisciplinary French consensus—part 1. J Cosmet Dermatol. 2011 Mar;10(1):36–50.
127. Bertossi D, Cavallini M, Cirillo P, Piero Fundarò S, Quartucci S, Sciuto C, Tonini D, Trocchi G, Signorini M. Italian consensus report on the aesthetic use of onabotulinum toxin A. J Cosmet Dermatol. 2018 Oct;17(5):719–730.
128. Cohen JL, Scuderi N. Safety and patient satisfaction of abobotulinumtoxin A for aesthetic use: a systematic review. Aesthet Surg J. 2017 May 1;37(suppl_1):S32–S44.
129. Carruthers J, Burgess C, Day D, Fabi SG, Goldie K, Kerscher M, Nikolis A, Pavicic T, Rho NK, Rzany B, Sattler G, Sattler S, Seo K, Werschler WP, Carruthers A. Consensus recommendations for combined aesthetic interventions in the face using botulinum toxin, fillers, and energy-based devices. Dermatol Surg. 2016 May;42(5):586–597.
130. Kane M, Donofrio L, Ascher B, Hexsel D, Monheit G, Rzany B, Weiss R. Expanding the use of neurotoxins in facial aesthetics: a consensus panel's assessment and recommendations. J Drugs Dermatol. 2010 Jan;9(1 Suppl):s7–22.
131. Raspaldo H, Baspeyras M, Bellity P, Dallara JM, Gassia V, Niforos FR, Belhaouari L, Consensus Group. Upper- and mid-face anti-aging treatment and prevention using onabotulinumtoxin A: the 2010 multidisciplinary French consensus—part 1. J Cosmet Dermatol. 2011 Mar;10(1):36–50.
132. Raspaldo H, Niforos FR, Gassia V, Dallara JM, Bellity P, Baspeyras M, Belhaouari L, Consensus Group. Lower-face and neck antiaging treatment and prevention using onabotulinumtoxin A: the 2010 multidisciplinary French consensus—part 2. J Cosmet Dermatol. 2011 Jun;10(2):131–149.
133. Zarringam D, Decates T, Slijper HP, Velthuis P. Increased usage of botulinum toxin and hyaluronic acid fillers in young adults. J Eur Acad Dermatol Venereol. 2020 Oct;34(10):e602–e604.
134. American Society for Aesthetic Plastic Surgery. Cosmetic (Aesthetic) surgery. National Data Bank STATISTICS. [Online]. Available at: www.surgery.org/sites/default/files/ASAPS-Stats2018_0.pdf.
135. Vance K, Howe W, Dellavalle RP. Social internet sites as a source of public health information. Dermatol Clin. 2009 Apr;27(2):133–136.

CHAPTER 2

Anatomy

CHAPTER 2.1

Surface Anatomy

Dario Bertossi and Ali Pirayesh

INTRODUCTION

The nasal shape is formed by the interplay of soft tissue structures with the underlying cartilaginous and bone framework. Variations of muscle, skin, cartilage, or bone **thickness** contribute to the surface anatomy. The profile on the nose, as well as its projection and ethnic features, are related to the **position and the shape** of the bony and cartilaginous structures caused by congenital, iatrogenic, or post-traumatic events. Anthropometric experts have reported classifications of nasal types using the shape of specific nasal details of different races to achieve shared defining characteristics [1,2].

When we examine a nose, we must first identify some common terms to describe the nasal areas, as we have to make records of the patient's defects and identify the points we can treat and those we should leave untreated in order to prevent further complications.

Second, we must identify the surrounding areas that may give us the chance to get the best result with the nose and select the proper material to be used in every area for a stable result.

Finally, we promote the use of a nasal grid to customize the treatment plan. Using this grid, and recording notes on the scheme eventually formulated, allows us to repeat the same treatment to achieve comparable results and make sure we perform a safe treatment.

NASAL TERMINOLOGY

On the **frontal view**, the nose is composed of a nasal base, where we can identify the two nostrils, two nasal alae, and a central portion which is the columella (see Figure 2.1.1). All these structures are linked to the upper maxilla that alongside with the pyriform aperture and the anterior nasal spine, hosts the facial muscles as well as the superficial and deep fat. The position and shape of the alar cartilages is influenced by the nasal septum, although these cartilages do not attach directly to the maxilla [3]. The crural cartilages [4–6] form the columella [6] (see Figure 2.1.2).

The upper part of the nasal base is the nasal tip, which is deeply supported by the alar cartilages and in the midline has the Pitanguy ligament as well as the nasal superficial muscular aponeurotic system (SMAS). The dermal-cartilaginous ligament of Pitanguy is retrievable in the medial portion of the nose and continues down to join both medial crura with the septum [3,4]. This ligament shapes the nasal tip as well as the interdomal fat pad [6–8].

As one proceeds up distally from the base, the nasal tip is followed by the nasal dorsum, which is supported in the midline by the nasal septum and the two paired triangular cartilages, as well as from the nasal bones (see Figure 2.1.3). The upper nose boundary is the glabella, which is between the two medial eye canthi (palpebral commissures) and connects the forehead and the nose itself. This area is supported by the frontal bone, the nasal bones, and the muscles below the skin and the superficial fat layer. Here we have the most important and crucial area for injections and surgery, which is bilaterally located on the nasal dorsum and glabella or nasion—the vascular network of the nasal dorsum (see Figure 2.1.4A and B).

On the **frontal and lateral view**, we can observe the following points (see Figure 2.1.5A and B):

Ans: Anterior nasal spine, showing the nasal labial angle projection resulting from the position of the anterior nasal spine, the thickness of the upper lip, and the columellar shape.
Rnb-Lnb: Right nasal base and left nasal base, showing the support of the piriform aperture and of the overlying muscles, fat, and skin.

SURFACE ANATOMY

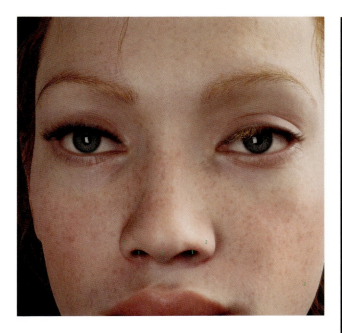

Figure 2.1.1 Nasal tip areas: 1 Alar rims; 2 Nasal alae; 3 Nasal columella.

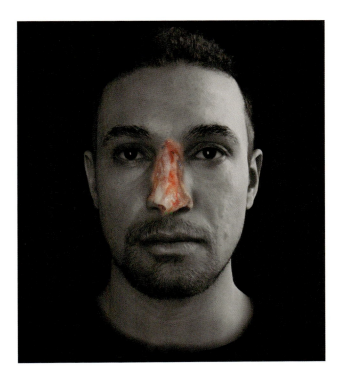

Figure 2.1.2 Medial cruras (green dots).

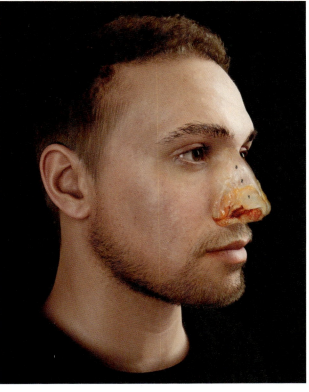

Figure 2.1.3 1 Right alar cartilage; 2 Right nasal cartilage; 3 Right nasal bone.

Itl: Infratip lobule, at the midpoint of the columella, supported by the medial cartilaginous cruras.
Nt: Nasal tip area, between the domes, the midportion of the crural cartilages.
Sta: Supratip area, a soft tissue area over the domes.
Tip defining points: Two points over the domes, showing the most apical area.
Nd: Nasal dorsum, starting over the domes and ending in the glabella.
G: Glabella, between the medial canthi of the eyes in the midpupillary line.

NASAL SURROUNDING AREAS

On the lateral view we can observe the same structures supporting the nasal soft tissues and therefore the shape, but we can better identify the surrounding areas that, when treated, may improve the nasal shape (see Figure 2.1.6).

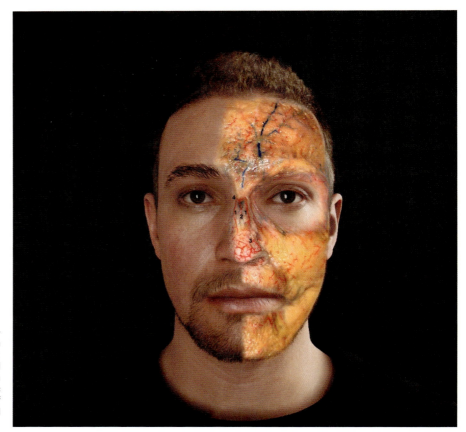

Figure 2.1.4A 1 Dorsal nasal arteries; 2 Middle branch on nasal dorsum; 3 Left lateral nasal artery; 4 Branch of the ophthalmic artery (branch of the internal carotid system).

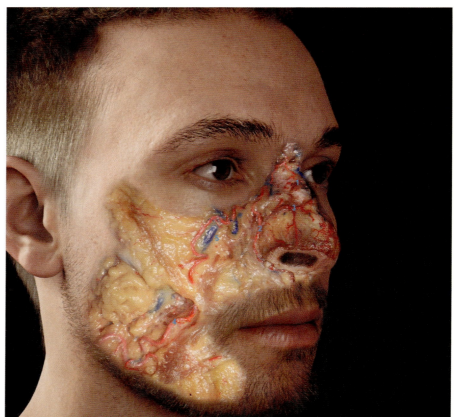

Figure 2.1.4B 1 Dorsal nasal artery; 2 Angular artery; 3 Left lateral nasal artery; 4 Right facial artery; 5 Right facial vein.

SURFACE ANATOMY

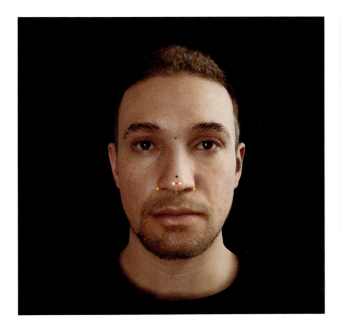

Figure 2.1.5A Nasal areas. **Ans** (green dot), anterior nasal spine; **Rnb-Lnb** (yellow dots), right nasal base and left nasal base; **Itl** (orange dot), infratip lobule; **Nt** (red dot), nasal tip area; **Sta** (blue dot), supratip area; **Tip defining points** (white dots), the dome's most apical area; **Nd** (gray line), nasal dorsum; **G** (purple dot), glabella.

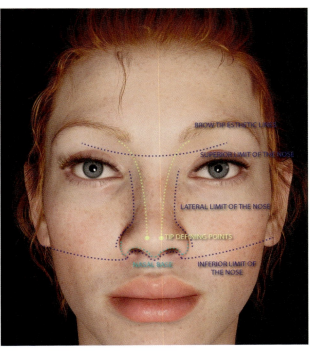

Figure 2.1.5B Nasal boundaries.

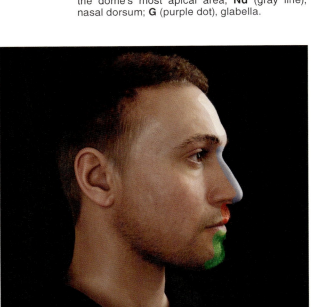

Figure 2.1.6 Nasal surrounding areas.

NASAL GRID

The grid is the reference for the quantity and sequence of injection records and allows reproducibility for future injections. Lines are traced onto a frontal view and a profile view (see Figures 2.1.7–2.1.8).

Vertical Lines

M (midline): Through point M (midline interpupillary) to point Sp (subnasal point)
A (nasal ala): Bilateral running through nasal ala insertion, parallel to M
S (on profile view): Line passing on the subnasale

Horizontal Lines

S: Through subnasale, perpendicular to line M
T: Through nasal tip, perpendicular to line M
St: Through supratip, perpendicular to line M
N: Through nasion, perpendicular to line M
I: Through intermediate between N and T, perpendicular to line M

LINES IDENTIFYING SPECIFIC POINTS

Na: Nasion
Nd: Nasal dorsum
St: Supratip
Nt: Nasal tip
Il: Infralobule on midline
Sn: Subnasale
Rnb: Right nasal bone area
Lnb: Left nasal bone area
Rna: Right nasal ala zone
Lna: Left nasal ala zone

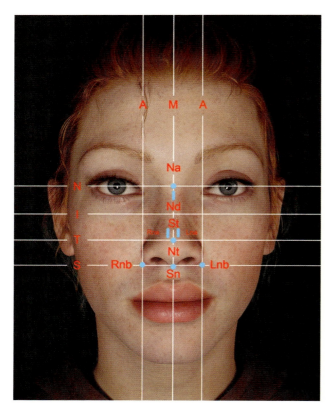

Figure 2.1.7 Frontal view of the nasal grid.

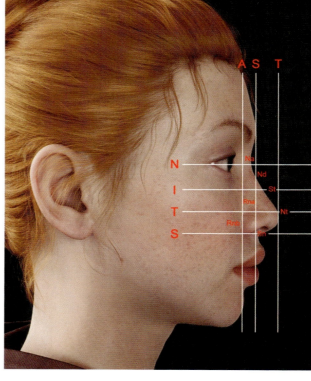

Figure 2.1.8 Side view of the nasal grid.

BIBLIOGRAPHY

1. Patel RG. Nasal anatomy and function. Facial Plast Surg. 2017 Feb;33(1):3–8.
2. Nguyen PS, Bardot J, Duron JB, et al. Anatomie chirurgicale de la pyramide nasale [Surgical anatomy of the nose]. Ann Chir Plast Esthet. 2014 Dec;59(6):380–386.
3. Oneal RM, Beil RJ, Jr, Schlesinger J. Surgical anatomy of the nose. Clin Plast Surg. 1996 Apr;23(2):195–222.
4. Galarza-Paez L, Marston G, Downs BW. Anatomy, head and neck, nose. In StatPearls [Internet]. Treasure Island (FL): StatPearls Publishing; 2021 Jul 26.
5. Henson B, Drake TM, Edens MA. Anatomy, head and neck, nose sinuses. In: StatPearls [Internet]. Treasure Island (FL): StatPearls Publishing; 2021 Jul 31.
6. AlJulaih GH, Sharma P, Lasrado S. Anatomy, head and neck, nose bones. In: StatPearls [Internet]. Treasure Island (FL): StatPearls Publishing; 2021 Aug 11.
7. Saban Y, Andretto Amodeo C, et al. An anatomical study of the nasal superficial musculoaponeurotic system: surgical applications in rhinoplasty. Arch Facial Plast Surg. 2008 Mar–Apr;10(2):109–115.
8. Anderson KJ, Henneberg M, Norris RM. Anatomy of the nasal profile. J Anat. 2008 Aug;213(2):210–216.

CHAPTER 2.2

Deep Anatomy

Dario Bertossi, Ali Pirayesh, Riccardo Nocini, and Andrea Sbarbati

The nose is a complex three-dimensional structure with a multiple-layer anatomy which must be evaluated before doing a nasal correction. Through an accurate description of the surface topography, we must observe its alternative concavities and convexities, which are influenced by the unique properties of the underlying tissues. The nose in fact possesses a rigid structural layer as well as an internal lining of cartilage and bone supporting the shape and function [1–9].

SKIN

In the upper third (glabella), the skin is thick and relatively distensible (flexible and mobile). It then tapers, becoming tightly adherent to the osteocartilaginous framework, thinning towards the dorsal nasal bridge. The middle third overlying the nasal bridge (mid-dorsal section) has the thinnest, most adherent, and least distensible skin. The skin of the lower third is of equal thickness to the upper nose, due to more sebaceous glands, especially at the nasal tip (see Figure 2.2.1).

FAT

The nose consists of a framework of skin, cartilage, and bone with six distinguishable layers (see Figure 2.2.2): skin, superficial fatty layer, fibromuscular layer (the superficial muscular aponeurotic system [SMAS]), deep fatty layer, periosteum, perichondrium, and bone cartilage. Nasal subcutaneous tissue exists in discrete compartments that are determined by the underlying perforator blood supply. The skin is thicker in the radix area. Immediately beneath the skin there is a superficial fatty layer comprising predominantly adipose tissue containing vertical fibers and septae extending from the skin to the underlying SMAS [8]. The distinct nasal SMAS is in continuation with the facial SMAS. Subcutaneous fat is concentrated in the glabella, lateral nasal wall, tip, and supratip areas. Distribution of the sub-SMAS fat is like

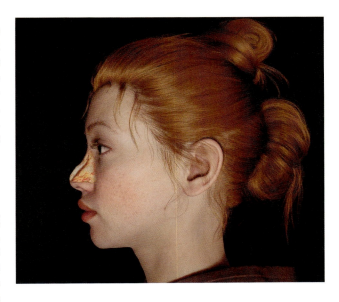

Figure 2.2.1 Elevated skin of the nasal area; observe the underlying nasal SMAS.

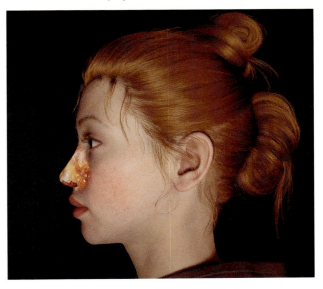

Figure 2.2.2 Nasal fat intermingled with the nasal SMAS.

that of the superficial facial fat with an additional layer of fat beneath the transverse nasalis muscle and the interdomal fat pad confirmed in cadaver studies.

MUSCLES

The nasal SMAS is a continuation of the facial SMAS. This layer unsheathes the muscles and is highly vascular. All the nasal muscles (see Figure 2.2.3) are innervated by the seventh cranial nerve. **Procerus**: The procerus is the most cephalic muscle of the nose. It arises from the glabellar area, extends caudally in a vertical fashion, and joins with the wing-shaped transverse nasalis muscle covering the caudal portion of the nasal bones. The main function of the procerus is depression of the eyebrows, which can create horizontal wrinkles over the cephalic portion of the nose in aging patients [9].

Nasalis: The nasal muscle has two components: the transverse nasalis or compressor nasi and the pars alaris. The transverse part of the muscle spans the dorsum of the nose, covering the upper lateral cartilages. This muscle, also called the pars-transversa, arises from the lateral cephalic portion of the sub-pyriform crescent. The pars-transversa joins with the procerus muscle and the opposite muscle in the midline to form the nasalis-procerus aponeurosis, which compresses and elongates the nose, contracts the nostrils, and narrows the vestibules. The second component of the nasalis muscle, the pars alaris (alar nasalis), arises from the crescent origin of the maxilla and is more lateral and slightly caudal to the bony origin of the depressor septi nasi muscle. The alar portion partially covers the lateral crus of the lower lateral cartilages and assists in dilatation of the nares. Damage to this muscle may result in collapse of the external nasal valve. In ethnic noses, the pars alaris is stronger and far more developed.

Depressor alae or myrtiforme: The depressor alae muscle originates from the border of the pyriform crest and then rises vertically, in a fanlike pattern, to the ala, acting as a depressor and constrictor of the nostrils.

Levator labii superioris alaeque nasi (LLSAN): The LLSAN plays an important functional role. It extends laterally to the nose in a cephalocaudal direction and has fibers that are attached to the nostrils, thus contributing to dilatation of the nares. Paralysis of these muscles will contribute to collapse of the external valve.

Depressor septi nasi: The depressor septi nasi arises from the maxilla just below the nasal spine, sometimes fuses with fibers of the orbicularis oris muscle, extends along the columellar base, and attaches to the foot plate. Occasionally fibers of this muscle extend to the middle genu. Some authors believe that these muscle fibers extend to the membranous septum. The depressor septi nasi depresses the nasal tip on animation and alters air turbulence. Additionally, it is of

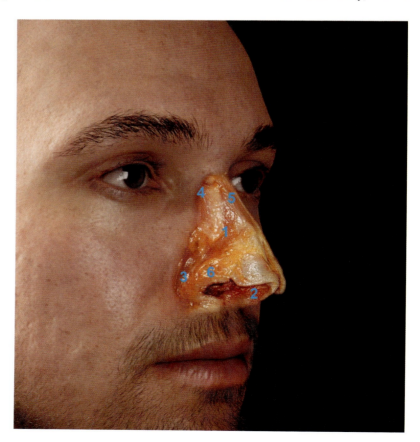

Figure 2.2.3 Nasal muscles: 1 Transverse nasalis; 2 Depressor septi nasi; 3 LANLS; 4 Depressor supracilii; 5 Procerus; 6 Dilator naris anterior.

DEEP ANATOMY

aesthetic importance, and its contraction narrows the labio-columellar angle. Release of this muscle not only eliminates the depressor effect on the tip but may also cause slight ptosis of the upper lip, which may or may not be beneficial, depending on the visibility of the patient's incisor teeth.

VASCULARIZATION

The arterial blood vessel supply to the nose is twofold: There is internal vascularization through branches of the internal carotid artery—a branch of the anterior ethmoidal artery, and a branch of the posterior ethmoid artery, which derive from the ophthalmic artery—and branches of the external carotid artery—the sphenopalatine artery and the greater palatine artery coming from the internal maxillary artery, the superior labial artery, and the angular artery coming from the facial artery. The latter becomes the angular artery in the proximity of the nasal ala and then courses over the superomedial aspect of the nose to become the lateral nasal artery (see Figure 2.2.4). The dorsal nose is supplied by branches of the internal maxillary artery (infraorbital) and the ophthalmic arteries, deriving from the internal carotid artery. This anastomotic area between the internal and external carotid circulations is very important, as it may lead to intravascular embolization of injected fillers (see Figure 2.2.5). The main branches form the columellar branches and the lateral nasal branches. The lateral nasal vessels are 2–3 mm above the alar groove, and, together with the columellar artery, arise deep at the nasal base to end at the tip in the subdermal plexus [16]; both supply the tip of the nose. Internally, the lateral nasal wall is supplied by the sphenopalatine artery

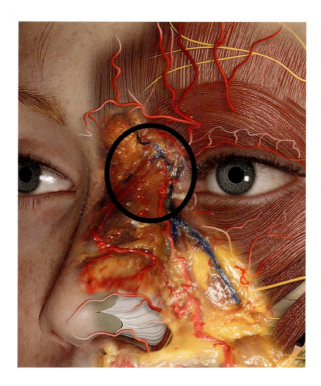

Figure 2.2.5 Anastomosis between internal and external carotid systems.

(from behind and below) and by the anterior and posterior ethmoid arteries (from above and behind). The nasal septum also is supplied by the sphenopalatine, anterior, and posterior ethmoid arteries, with additional contribution by the superior labial and greater palatine arteries. These three vascular supplies to the internal nose converge in the Kiesselbach plexus (Little's area), a region in the anteroinferior third of the nasal septum. Furthermore, the venous supply of the nose generally follows the arterial pattern of nasal vascularization. The nasal veins are biologically significant because they have no valves and communicate directly with the cavernous sinus. This may cause intracranial spread of bacterial infections originating from the nasal region. Intra-arterial injections in this area may lead to skin necrosis and even blindness. Danger zones exist, particularly in the areas where the internal and external carotid systems communicate (angular artery and columellar artery). Due to great anatomic variability, the midline position as a safe reference may sometimes be unsafe for injection. Therefore, we emphasize the principle of "staying deep," just above the periosteum and perichondrium.

INNERVATION

Nasal sensory innervation is derived from the supraorbital and infraorbital nerves; motor innervation is via the buccal branch of the facial nerve (see Figure 2.2.6).

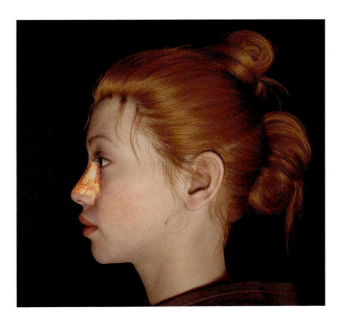

Figure 2.2.4 Anatomy of the nasal vascularization.

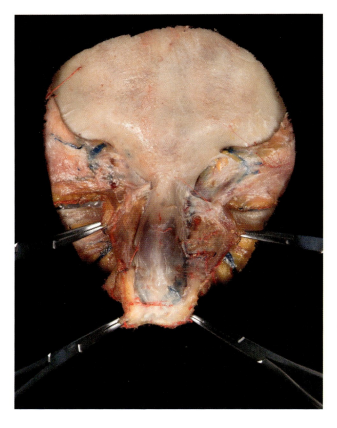

Figure 2.2.6 Supratrochlear and supraorbital nerves.

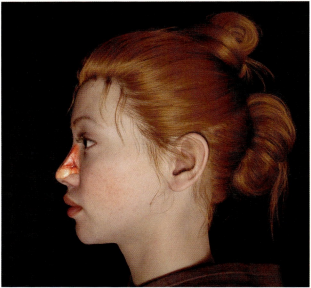

Figure 2.2.7 Nasal bones and cartilages.

BONE

The skeletal component of the nose consists of bone and cartilage (see Figure 2.2.7). The paired nasal bones and the frontal process of the maxilla form the lateral aspect, whilst the lateral surfaces of the upper two-thirds join in the midline at the nasal dorsum. Superolaterally the paired nasal bones connect to the lacrimal bones, and inferolaterally they attach to the ascending processes of the maxilla. Posterosuperiorly, the bony nasal septum is composed of the perpendicular plate of the ethmoidal bone. The vomer lies posteroinferiorly and partially forms the choanal opening into the nasopharynx. The nasal floor is formed by the pre-maxillary and the palatine bones, which also form the roof of the mouth. The bony nasal vault comprises the paired nasal bones and the ascending frontal process of the maxilla. This part of the nose is pyramidal in shape, the narrowest portion being at the intercanthal line. The average length of the nasal bone is 25 mm, although there may be both individual and significant ethnic variation (African American noses often have short nasal bones). Laterally the nasal bones join with the frontal process of the maxilla. The circle created with the nasal spine, the thin portion of the frontal process of the maxilla, and the thin caudal border of the nasal bones is called the pyriform aperture. The nasal bones fuse with the superior edge of the perpendicular plate of the ethmoid bone cephalad to the intercanthal line. The confluence of cartilaginous nasal septum, ethmoid bone, and nasal bone is called the keystone area.

CARTILAGE

The cartilaginous nasal frame consists of a pair of upper and lower lateral cartilages and the nasal septum (see Figure 2.2.8). The upper lateral cartilages are paired rectangular cartilages that support the lateral nasal walls. These cartilages join the septum in the midline, although the fusion between the upper lateral cartilages and the septum occurs in a manner which almost creates a single unit cephalically. The lateral border of the upper lateral cartilages frequently terminates at the level of the lateral nasal bone suture line. This leaves a space between the bone and upper lateral cartilage, which is termed the external lateral triangle. It is surrounded by the caudal border of the upper lateral cartilages cephalically, the frontal process of the maxilla laterally, and the cephalic border of the lower lateral cartilage caudally. The cephalic portion of the upper lateral cartilage is overlapped by the nasal bone. The amount of overlap is highly variable and can range from 2 to 11 mm.

The lower lateral cartilages have four components: the medial crus, middle crus, dome, and lateral crus. The medial crus has two distinct segments: the footplate and the columella. The footplate varies in size and in the degree of lateral angulation. This angulation of the

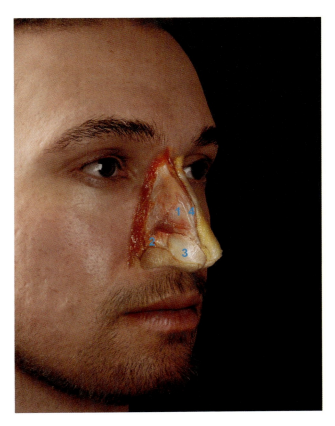

Figure 2.2.8 1 Right lateral cartilage; 2 Sesamoid cartilages; 3: Right lateral crus; 4 Nasal septum.

footplate governs the width of the base of the columella. The columellar segment of the medial crus varies in length and width; the longer the columellar portion, the longer the nostril and thus the potential for a more projected nasal tip. Cephalad to this portion of the medial crura is the membranous septum, which is composed of two layers of soft tissues encasing some fibrous bands named septo-columellar ligaments. The middle crus, part of the lower lateral cartilage, extends between the medial crus and the domes, and its length and width largely control the configuration of the infratip lobule. The domal segment is the narrowest and thinnest portion of the lower lateral cartilage, yet it is the most important in relation to the tip shape. There is tremendous variation in its shape; on rare occasions, it has a convolution that, when present, invariably results in bulbosity of the tip. The area posterior and caudal to the domes, between the medial and lateral segments, contains two segments of soft tissue, with no cartilage, is externally covered with skin and internally with the vestibular lining, and is called the soft triangle. The medial and middle crura are tightly bound together by fibrous bands. The most anterior one is called the interdomal ligament. Additionally, there are fibrous bands more anteriorly binding the domes to each other and the overlying dermis; these are called the Pitanguy ligament. There are additional fibrous bands at the level of the footplates and between the upper and lower lateral cartilages.

The lateral crus is the largest component of the nasal lobule. It is narrow anteriorly but becomes wider in the midportion and narrows again laterally. The lateral crus of the lower lateral cartilage are usually in contact with the first chain of the accessory cartilages that abut the pyriform aperture. Medially, the lateral crus are continuous with the domal segment. The anterior portion of this cartilage can curve in a variety of directions and controls the convexity of the ala. It also provides support to the anterior half of the alar rim. However, posteriorly, it diverges and does not have much contribution to the ala, yet does contribute to the function of the external valve. Generally, this cartilage is oriented at a 45-degree angle to the vertical facial plane. The curled junction of the cephalic edge of the lateral crus and the caudal edge of the upper lateral cartilage is referred to as the scroll area. The magnitude of curling can vary from patient to patient and is sometimes significant enough to cause external visibility and fullness in this area. The lower lateral cartilage is commonly short and weak in non-Caucasian noses. The accessory cartilages are a series of small cartilages situated on the nasal ala close to the tail of the alar cartilages. The nasal septum is situated on the central part of the nose, and it's connected with its inferior surface with the upper maxillary crest, the posterior and the anterior nasal spine, and is connected to the nasal bones in the key area where the two upper lateral cartilages are also connected to it, forming the internal nasal valve.

BIBLIOGRAPHY

1. Patel RG. Nasal anatomy and function. Facial Plast Surg. 2017 Feb;33(1):3–8.
2. Nguyen PS, Bardot J, Duron JB, et al. Anatomie chirurgicale de la pyramide nasale [Surgical anatomy of the nose]. Ann Chir Plast Esthet. 2014 Dec;59(6):380–386.
3. Oneal RM, Beil RJ Jr, Schlesinger J. Surgical anatomy of the nose. Clin Plast Surg. 1996 Apr;23(2):195–222.
4. Galarza-Paez L, Marston G, Downs BW. Anatomy, head and neck, nose. In StatPearls [Internet]. Treasure Island (FL): StatPearls Publishing; 2021 Jul 26.
5. Henson B, Drake TM, Edens MA. Anatomy, head and neck, nose sinuses. In StatPearls [Internet]. Treasure Island (FL): StatPearls Publishing; 2021 Jul 31.
6. AlJulaih GH, Sharma P, Lasrado S. Anatomy, head and neck, nose bones. In StatPearls [Internet]. Treasure Island (FL): StatPearls Publishing; 2021 Aug 11.
7. Sobiesk JL, Munakomi S. Anatomy, head and neck, nasal cavity. In StatPearls [Internet]. Treasure Island (FL): StatPearls Publishing; 2021 Jul 26.
8. Han SK, Shin YW, Kim WK. Anatomy of the external nasal nerve. Plast Reconstr Surg. 2004 Oct;114(5):1055–1059.
9. Konschake M, Fritsch H. Anatomical mapping of the nasal muscles and application to cosmetic surgery. Clin Anat. 2014 Nov;27(8):1178–1184.

CHAPTER **3**

Clinical Aspects

CHAPTER **3.1**

Clinical Defects and the Technical Approach

Woodrow Wilson and Dario Bertossi

INTRODUCTION TO THE TECHNICAL DEVICES FOR HIGHLIGHTING AND REPORTING CLINICAL DEFECTS: PHOTOGRAPHY AND OPTICAL IMAGING

Surgeons and physicians engaged in plastic surgery and aesthetic medicine should rely on a scientific objective and accurate imaging data of patients undergoing the treatment, just starting from optical photography [1]. There are three technological pathways for capturing clinical photography—traditional two-dimensional (2D) using a digital single lens reflex (DSLR), three-dimensional (3D) surface imaging or augmented reality. 3D imaging has come to have a big impact on aesthetic surgery worldwide [1,2]. The first attempt to use the 3D surface imaging technique in a clinic dates to 1944 by Thalmaan, who used stereo photogrammetry to examine an adult with facial asymmetry and a baby with Pierre Robin syndrome.

Since then, photography for aesthetic medicine evolved, and 3D photography has become greatly used, allowing for a more dynamic facial evaluation, although it is associated with an increased cost [3,4]. Accurate 2D imaging as a lower-cost entry point has been pursued [13]. Doctors approaching either plastic surgery or non-surgical rhinoplasty or profileplasty should be ensured of the soundness and high-quality outcome of patients' photos, as the advantages of a high sharpness in the visual result of a photo allow the surgeon to screen and detect any small defects on the face skin and anatomy, enabling him or her to plan a correct surgical or non-surgical intervention [5]. The principles outlined in this chapter allow for accurate capture of the nose, but also the entire face, mandible and neckline.

Standardization helps surgeons to evaluate their own procedures and postoperative outcomes, thus reducing many complex variables that could taint the overall result of the whole process [6]. Accurate clinical photography of the patient is integral to the consultation process, patient understanding and increasingly generating education and advertising collateral for the clinician or practice.

Furthermore, the increasing trend of patients understanding their anatomy through mobile phones (selfies) and social media needs to be considered. These interpretations need to be balanced by the clinician upon baseline image capture so as to identify anatomical distortions and/or body dysmorphia caused by technological biases such as optical distortion, software skin filtering or proportion manipulation [16,17].

In the technical approach using photography, a difference between understanding the syntactic and semantic structure of a single picture and understanding the "language" of a combination of more than one image must be identified [6]. Two kinds of classification can be superimposed: a) First, a series of photographs deals with a theme, for example, a series about Yosemite National Park. The order of the photos is not significant and can be created by the photographer. b) Second, a sequence of photographs tells us a visual story. c) Third, a timeline of the photography exhibits a change over time regarding the same subject within a defined interval. It is obvious that both medical and aesthetic photographic documentation falls into this latter category by demonstrating changes in body surface and/or contour in each time frame after a medical/aesthetic treatment or procedure [6].

To create a timeline in the photography, all photos' conditions should preferably be still to recognize modifications in the subject, which has been properly documented. These circumstances are bullet pointed in terms of camera calibration, distance between the photo operator and the patient, the perspective/angle of the camera, background brightness and color, picture sizing and pixeling and finally, lighting.

Modern cameras are in fact miniature computer devices with an imaging sensor, and so can be calibrated for reproducible results [13]. Understanding the theoretical principles of shutter, aperture and sensor sensitivity is recommended, but not essential, to the clinician once the camera is programmed. This is often a barrier that inhibits clinicians from pursuing accurate clinical photography. Instead, the focus should be placed on correct alignment of the camera and positioning of the patient in static and dynamic sequences.

Modern digital cameras have many software novelties, which can create an image once it is already revised by the same software. On the other hand, two different cameras will result in two different representations of the same subject/reality, thereby reducing the accuracy of the photographic documentation. Moreover, maintaining a fixed perspective or angle is paramount to reproducible aesthetic photographic documentation. The way in which the camera is set should be at a comparable level as the individual of her or his anatomic appearance and area. Obviously, this means that the camera moves upward to screen the face and downwards if screening the knees. Our camera should remain in a fixed X plane; however, the Y plane will adjust according to patient height. The lens barrel should be parallel to the floor (Y) and perpendicular to the image sensor.

Background color, light, brightness and sharpness should remain constant in a photographic timeline. The distortion potential of brightness and colors was already demonstrated by cognitive psychology in the 1940s. For medical and aesthetic photographic documentation, gray or dark blue backgrounds are recommended. These backgrounds provide the clearest separation between the background and subject, regardless of the Fitzpatrick scale of the subject's skin (see Figure 3.1.1).

Backgrounds can either be a pull-down banner blind or painted wall. A painted wall using matte paint as opposed to glossy limits reflections.

Most modern cameras have an integrated flash; however, this is not powerful enough to expose our subject correctly and should be avoided. A clinical photography area requires dedicated flash strobe lighting separate from the camera. A strobe light emits a pulse of light which simulates sunlight at noon (5500K) with a typical T.1 (time taken for 90% of flash power to be emitted) of 1/1000th of a second.

The speed of this pulse has the additional benefit of freezing the subject without the use of a tripod and, combined with correct camera calibration, nullifying the ambient light dictated by time-of-day variation or overhead lighting.

This infrastructure also ensures accurate color of patient skin, showcasing changes in radiance and reflection. It also illuminates the background behind the patient, eliminating the need for a second light dedicated to the background.

There are two clear schools of thought regarding lighting, one being the use of a single light (see Figure 3.1.2a), and the other two lights (see Figure 3.1.2b).

The fundamental objective of introducing a light source is to ensure consistency of exposure, angle of light and color of light regardless of the time of day or interval between capture sessions. Second, it is important to

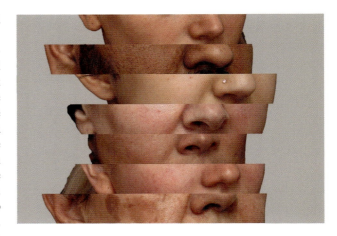

Figure 3.1.1 Fitzpatrick scale of a patient's skin type.

represent the human face in a natural way (so as to have the patient recognize themselves) by not introducing artificial shadowing in key parts of the face.

A single light source at a fixed distance from the patient ensures the exposure does not change. Given the power of a strobe light at 400w, we need to factor in diffusion of the light source.

Another clear advantage of using a single light is the ability to use the clinical room itself as a diffusion source, which in turn alleviates the floor space required by two light sources [13]. A singular light source placed 180 cm (including allocating distance for reflected light) above the patient will create a reflected light angle of 45 degrees from the ceiling. Two light sources are placed 150 cm away at 45 degrees to the patient (see Figure 3.1.3).

Two lights can introduce artificial shadowing—for example, exaggerated shadows in the nasolabial fold (NLF), tear trough and nasal tip (see Figure 3.1.4). Much the same as optical distortion, we are introducing a bias that can affect the representation of the anatomy in a false manner. A single light will also create a more 3D overall shadow profile in the image.

PATIENT PREPARATION

With regard to the patient's preparation, all makeup and jewelry must be removed for all photographic documentation, including the posttreatment pictures. Briefly speaking, photographs used in pretreatment without makeup and posttreatment photographs with makeup must be fully avoided.

During each photographic session the patient should be clear of distractions and skin products. Specifically, makeup, sun care products or moisturizer needs to be removed. Adherence is essential, as these variations can alter the facial contours, proportions and skin reflectivity—which can negate the treatment result.

CLINICAL DEFECTS AND THE TECHNICAL APPROACH

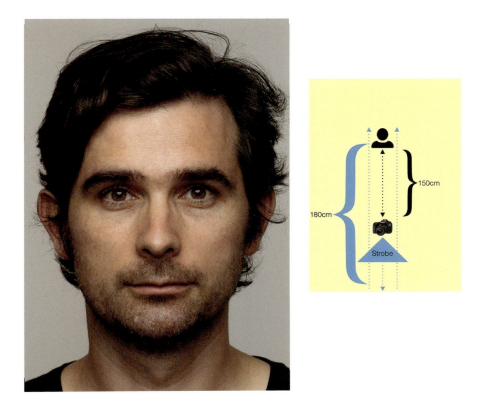

Figure 3.1.2a The use of a single light for a patient's pictures.

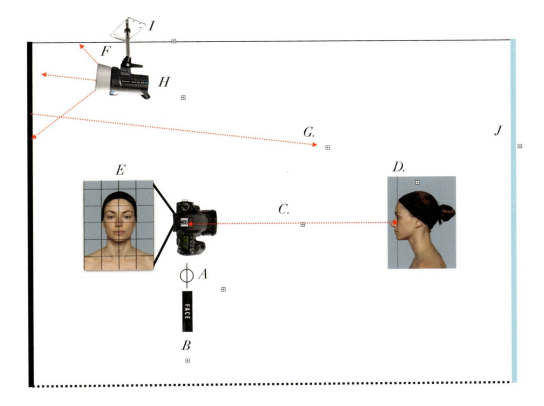

Figure 3.1.2b The use of a double light for a patient's pictures.

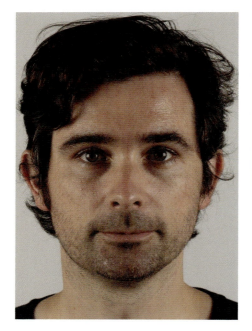
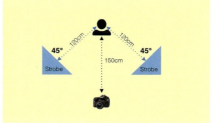

Figure 3.1.3 Two light sources placed 150 cm away at 45 degrees to the patient.

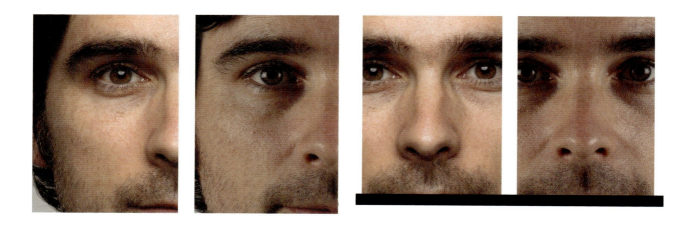

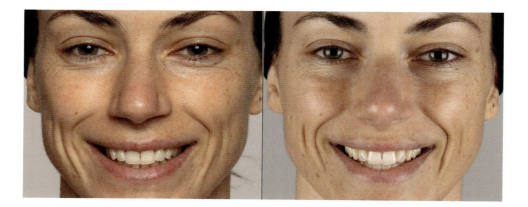

Figure 3.1.4a-c Two lights can introduce artificial shadowing—for example, exaggerated shadows in the NLF, tear trough and nasal tip.

In the case of patients wearing glasses, it is possible to take a photograph either with or without glasses, whereas scarves or hats must be removed. For the body, photographing the body mandates a decision regarding inclusion of undergarments in the pictures. When optical conditions occur, the patient may ask to be photographed in the absence of undergarments. Anyway, as this is not always practicable and forbidden in certain cultures, the surgeon should take an agreed decision. The minimum requirement to ensure consistent photographic documentation is that the patient wears the same undergarments of his or her choosing in all photographs. Photos must provide the best impression even for an external, not engaged subject or observer. To accomplish this goal, the clinic or office team (all members of the staff involved in photographic documentation) must be trained in the photographic and medical standards for achieving comparable photos—we mean a sound and meaningful deal of documents of what resulted as evidence from the procedures, even when compared with the previous clinical situation. Attempts to adjust and compensate for unexpected variability may be allowed to get a standardized imaging, even using some available editing software. Although today some companies (Canfield; Quantificare, Canada; Fotofinder, Germany, Adobe Lightroom USA) have developed new automatic units for 3D and 2D photographic documentation, thorough knowledge of the basic photographic standards is essential.

EQUIPMENT

Camera selection is vital; however, an agnostic approach to brands is important. As previously stated, modern cameras are essentially computers, so settings can be programmed into any brand such as Sony, Canon, Nikon, Leika, Contax, Hasselblad or Olympus. Each has appropriate lens and sensor combinations.

The specific in imaging resolution are important, and a 24-megapixel (mpx), APS-C sized imaging sensor and user-programmable profiles should be selected at a minimum. The higher the resolution, the more detail captured, and future proofing the image use pipeline. The use of a high-resolution camera of 24 mpx allows for a single image to be captured and then cropped down in postproduction according to the desired area required (see Figure 3.1.5).

Lens selection is an important factor, and a focal length between 75mm and 100mm (in 35mm terms) is recommended.

Once correct camera settings are programmed [13], the clinician can focus on the appropriate angles and techniques. There is a trifecta of settings that are required to work in unison with the strobe flash, namely, the speed of image capture (shutter), the amount of light allowed through the lens and onto the sensor (aperture) and the sensitivity of the sensor itself (ISO).

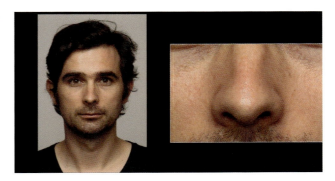

Figure 3.1.5 The use of a high-resolution camera of 24 mpx allows for a single image to be captured and then cropped down in postproduction according to the desired area required.

A shutter speed of between 1/125 and 1/160 is recommended to further negate the ambient light; an aperture value of between f11 and f13 to capture sufficient depth of field; and a sensor sensitivity of 100 to maximize color, detail, and noise fidelity. Fine-tuning these values to achieve optical exposure is key, then once attained, locked permanently to a user camera profile.

FRAMING TECHNIQUE

Regardless of the initial treatment enquiry—surgical or non-surgical—it is imperative that both static and dynamic images are captured at baseline consultation. The human face is a dynamic area, and patients may not be fully aware of their asymmetry, profile views or degree of movement. Dynamic expressions should be done in the anterior view at a minimum, and if time permits, at profile and three-quarters. This is a technique to thoroughly explain to a patient their own anatomy, but also to protect the clinician in case of disagreement on outcome.

Enabling a standard 6 × 4 cell grid on your camera allows you to see framing guidelines. We recommend the Frankfort plane alignment with the center frame line. By aligning the central frame line with the Frankfort line, you can solve several problems in your framing—namely camera-to-subject distance, perspective and height. In conjunction with the studio flash strobe properties previously described, this eliminates the need for a tripod.

As the camera has a built-in spirit level, you will be able to see if your patient needs to raise or lower their chin in the sagittal (X plane) relative to the Frankfort plane.

Start by capturing the patient profile right, with patient looking to their left, which allows you to calibrate with the Frankfort plane, then rotate patient in 45-degree increments. Ensure the patient rotates the head, hips and feet and not just their head.

Do not change your x- or y-axis by holding your camera still or being assisted by a tripod.

PICTURE PROTOCOL

1. Patient arrives at the clinic and fills out a form with all the data and the requested information regarding the defect and expectations.
2. Patient removes jewelry and makeup, moisture or sunscreen.
3. Patient wears a black-labeled tee shirt and a black hair band.
4. Patient is positioned in the rotating platform (see Diagram 3.1.1) and makes the following pictures:

- Front (see Figure 3.1.6)

Then a short video with the same facial expressions is taken (see Video 3.1.1. Available at https://resourcecentre.routledge.com/books/9781032303444).

The patient position must be assessed accurately to prevent common mistakes (see Figure 3.1.12. Available at https://resourcecentre.routledge.com/books/9781032303444). At the end of the session the pictures must be mounted in a PowerPoint or a Keynote file with the aid of facial lines (see Figures 3.1.13 and 3.1.14. Available at https://resourcecentre.routledge.com/books/9781032303444) to get a patient history available during the clinical consultation.

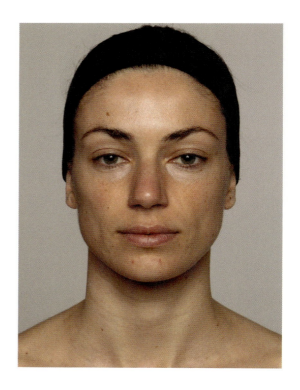

Figure 3.1.6 Front view of the patient.

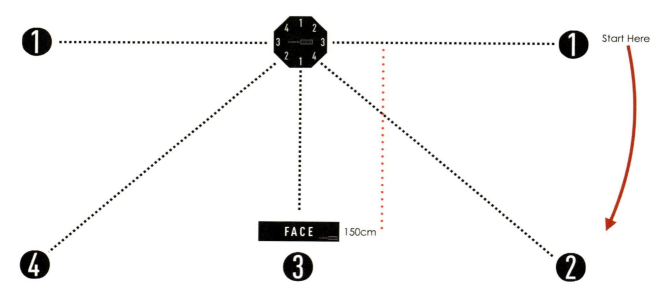

Diagram 3.1.1 Patient positions.

CLINICAL DEFECTS AND THE TECHNICAL APPROACH

- Left and right profiles (see Figure 3.1.7 a and b)

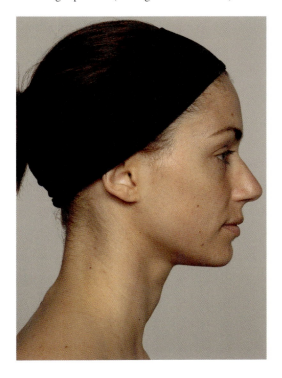

Figure 3.1.7a Right profile view of the patient.

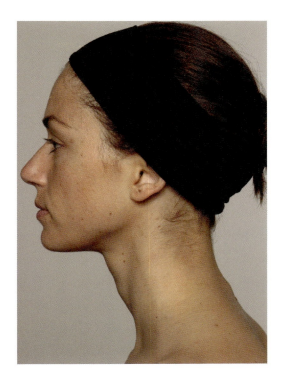

Figure 3.1.7b Left profile view of the patient.

- Left and right three-quarters (see Figure 3.1.8 a and b)

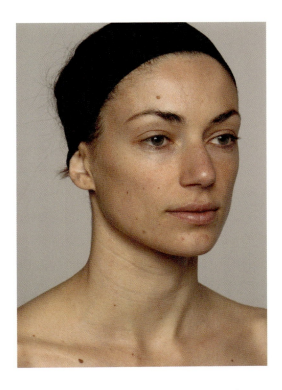

Figure 3.1.8a Right three-quarters view of the patient.

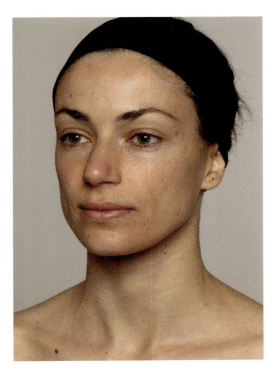

Figure 3.1.8b Left three-quarters view of the patient.

- Below view (see Figure 3.1.9)
- Above view (see Figure 3.1.10)

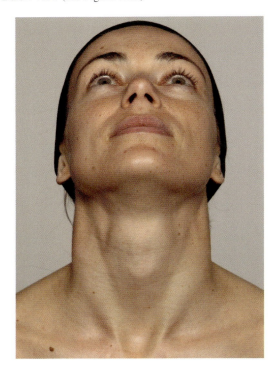

Figure 3.1.9   Below view of the patient.

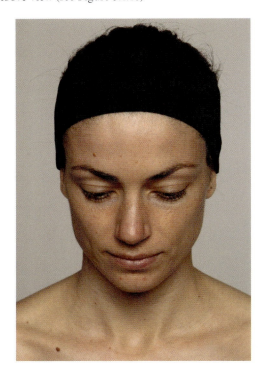

Figure 3.1.10   Above view of the patient.

- Same pictures with smile, frown, kissing, surprised and crying expressions (see Figure 3.1.11 a–e).

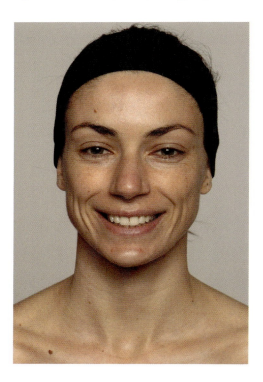

Figure 3.1.11a   Front view of the patient with a smile.

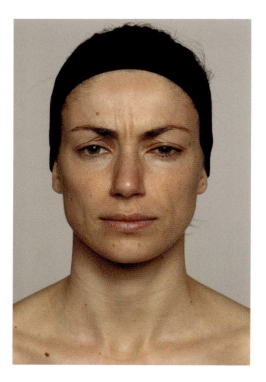

Figure 3.1.11b   Front view of the patient with a frown.

CLINICAL DEFECTS AND THE TECHNICAL APPROACH

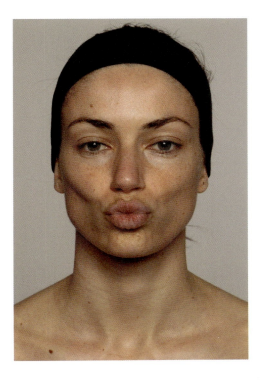

Figure 3.1.11c Front view of the patient with a kissing expression.

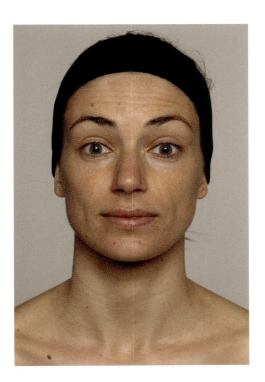

Figure 3.1.11d Front view of the patient with a surprised expression.

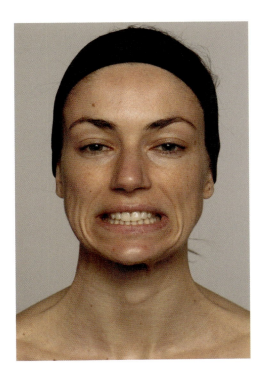

Figure 3.1.11e Front view of the patient with a crying expression.

BIBLIOGRAPHY

1. Mueller GP, Khan HA, Frame JD. New horizons in imaging and diagnosis in rhinoplasty. Oral Maxillofac Surg Clin North Am. 2021 Feb;33(1):1–5.
2. Lin SW, Sutherland K, Liao YF, Cistulli PA, Chuang LP, Chou YT, Chang CH, Lee CS, Li LF, Chen NH. Three-dimensional photography for the evaluation of facial profiles in obstructive sleep apnoea. Respirology. 2018 Jun;23(6):618–625.
3. Markiewicz MR, Bell RB. The use of 3D imaging tools in facial plastic surgery. Facial Plast Surg Clin North Am. 2011 Nov;19(4):655–682.
4. Tzou CH, Frey M. Evolution of 3D surface imaging systems in facial plastic surgery. Facial Plast Surg Clin North Am. 2011 Nov;19(4):591–602.
5. Schendel SA, Duncan KS, Lane C. Image fusion in preoperative planning. Facial Plast Surg Clin North Am. 2011 Nov;19(4):577–590.
6. Prantl L, Brandl D, Ceballos P. A proposal for updated standards of photographic documentation in aesthetic medicine. Plast Reconstr Surg Glob Open. 2017 Aug 17;5(8):e1389.
7. Henderson JT, Mullens CL, Woodberry KM. US public's perceptions of online transformation photos. Aesthet Surg J. 2021 Nov 12;41(12):1483–1491.

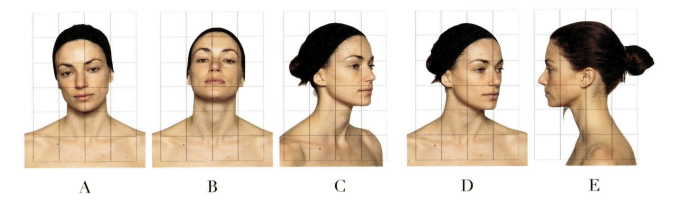

Figure 3.1.12 Mistakes taking pictures.

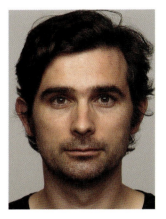 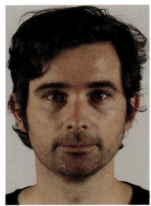 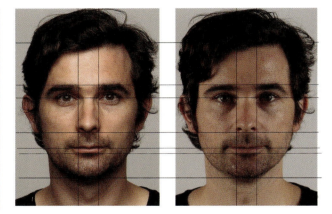

Figure 3.1.13 Pre- and post-treatment pictures in a PowerPoint file.

Figure 3.1.14 Pre- and post-treatment pictures in a PowerPoint file.

8. A standardised system of photography to assess cosmetic facial surgery. Available at: https://ajops.com/index.php/ajops/article/download/334/506/5250.
9. www.schorsch.com/en/kbase/glossary/cct.html.
10. Nasal distortion in short-distance photographs: the selfie effect.
11. www.ncbi.nlm.nih.gov/pmc/articles/PMC5876805/.
12. Selfies: living in the era of filtered photographs. Available at: https://doi.org/10.1001/jamafacial.2018.0486.
13. Predictors of acceptance of cosmetic surgery: Instagram images-based activities, appearance comparison and body dissatisfaction among women. Available at: www.researchgate.net/publication/354342252_Predictors_of_Acceptance_of_Cosmetic_Surgery_Instagram_Images-_Based_Activities_Appearance_Comparison_and_Body_Dissatisfaction_Among_Women.
14. Six-position, frontal view photography in blepharoplasty: a simple method. Available at: https://link.springer.com/article/10.1007/s00266-018-1104-3.

CHAPTER 3.2

Patient Consultation

Dario Bertossi and Ali Pirayesh

The medical consultation is the most important part of our work and represents the first moment of contact with the patient. At this stage, the patient feels vulnerable, and listening carefully to them is a way to understand who they are and how they see and feel about themselves. At this stage it is crucial to build the most important aspect of the patient-doctor relationship: **TRUST**.

This stage in our "treatment protocols" focuses on three important points:

1. **LISTEN**: We should never interrupt the patient who is talking about **why** she or he is coming to us. A minimum of 45 seconds listening is the key to understand the feelings of the patient and how she or he relates to the nasal defect. This individual is talking to us because of a sentence he heard about his defect, a face he saw in his mirror in the morning, a dream he had looking at the media identifying a symbol or a face she or he would love to match.
2. **OBSERVE**: While we listen to our patients, we should always observe the nose and its features relative to the face because the next step will be addressing them in front of the mirror, uncovering the real problems which normally are not visible to the patient. The consultation is focused primarily on patient education, as the main barriers are usually a lack of understanding of facial harmony, concerns over an unnatural outcome and side effects. Another key aspect of the first consultation is to reassure patients with appropriate words that our goal is not to change their face, but rather to emphasize their beauty while always maintaining their personality and uniqueness.
3. **PLAN:** Here the correct use of language is essential. Putting patients at ease at this stage is central to ensuring that they will return for treatment. Every face is different and complex, and hence, it is difficult to completely standardize the approach. With the use of professional pictures and a mirror (see Figure 3.2.1), we must customize a treatment plan following the anatomy of the face, identify the points and specify the amount of filler to be injected. Once these are identified we take notes on digital documents with dedicated illustrations (see Figure 3.2.2) with which we will be able to inform the patient about the costs of the treatment. In our daily practice we established a fixed cost for a non-surgical rhinoplasty. This means that we may use one or two syringes to deliver the best result. If the patient needs corrections in the surrounding areas, the cost will be calculated according to the needed points and amount of filler.

After these three very important points, we must describe accurately and with simple language the possible complications. These include obstruction of one of the branches of the ophthalmic artery, as well as eventual consequences such as clots or infection, and delayed complications like

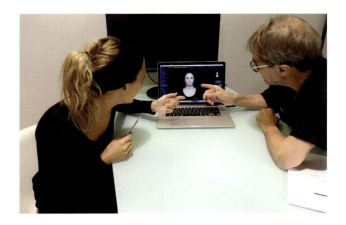

Figure 3.2.1 The accurate use of professional pictures and a mirror can give the patient the proper impression of their real aesthetic defects.

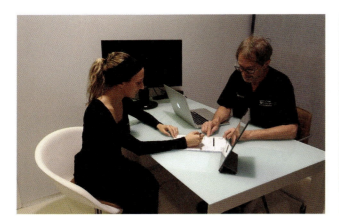

Figure 3.2.2 Paper and digital documents with proper illustrations showing the patient our possible treatment plan.

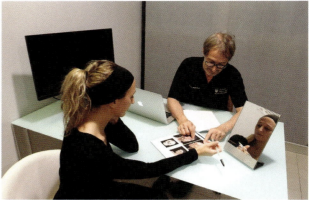

Figure 3.2.3 The correct anatomy description with paper and digital documentation shows the patient the possible complications.

swelling or nodules must be elucidated precisely. Bruising is the most frequent event because the nose has a very rich vascular network. Among this the anastomosis between the external and internal carotid systems on the nasal dorsum and glabellar area makes this area risky for the worst biological damage, which is blindness (see Chapter 9 and Figure 3.2.3).

Before we conclude the consultation, which normally should last between 10 minutes and 1 hour, we should keep in mind that rushing into an immediate treatment may give the patient the impression that you fear losing income. Most of the times, we prefer to give a patient the chance to go home and think about what has been discussed and reflect on our treatment plan and the possible complications or the eventual questions that may pop up in a familiar environment such as their home. Those who will come back are the ones in which you will have built the TRUST.

Be sincere, show confidence and be constantly logical with the support of science. These things are understood and felt by anyone.

Discover and enhance each individual feature that brings beauty in everyone's face. This is the secret for a patient's happiness, which is not a duty, but a wish.

MD CODES

An unexpected event, which may occur, regards patients undergoing an aesthetic procedure and resulting in a dissatisfied outcome [1–3]. In this circumstance, often patients focus their unhappy consideration onto defined facial areas, for example, jowls or periorbital area, thus asking surgeons to provide a better-suited revision [4–8]. Patients may be also dissatisfied in terms of outcome beyond the removal of isolated flaws, despite the successful action of hyaluronic acid (HA) fillers. They usually hope for a global assessment of their facial appearance, such as a more relaxed, cheerful or less tired or aged look, following any treatment [9].

However, facial appearance may convey a huge deal of different emotional messages or cues, and often they may not reflect the subject's real feeling, as occurring if a tired face may look as such even if a patient is not tired or a face may resemble sadness even if the patient is never sad [9–14]. Approaching a beautiful face with aesthetic medicine should encompass both a global overview of the face and the psychological attitude or orientation of the subject.

Interestingly, many investigations have assessed that many negative emotional inputs can be associated with facial deficiencies [9–11,13,15]. This may occur, for example, from glabellar lines that can convey the appearance of an angry face or for eye bags, letting the patient look tired [10,11,13,15].

Any of these negative emotional messages may come from changes mainly due to aging, involving skin, soft tissues and bones [9,11,13].

And yet, the treatment of a single area of the face, eye bags, for example, may not result in an overall beautiful facial appearance, so that several authors introduced in their aesthetic approaches even emotional messages (as mimic codes) or miscues of the subject's facial look [9,10,15]. These authors experienced that satisfaction occurred in patients when emotional messages were addressed, rather than considering isolated facial areas.

As a great deal of facial expression, i.e., happiness, sadness, fear, anger, fatigue and so on, do exist, these ones can be grouped and classified to match them with aesthetic approaches and finally improve the aesthetic techniques [9,13,15]. For example, it is possible to gather different cases into at least four favorable subgroups, such as looking attractive, younger, more contoured, and feminine or soft for females and masculine for males.

Notwithstanding, addressing what we recognize as unfavorable facial attributes is challenging, as a substantial number of variables can occur and may interfere with a successful outcome. Moreover, variables exist, such as age, ethnicity, and gender, which cannot be modified and included in the surgeon's control. What is very interesting is that any of these features may affect facial anatomy, such as fat content, muscle function and activity, skin laxity, hydration and quality, thus resulting in an enormous collection of "different faces", thus influencing also the way by which filler injections should be accomplished. For these reasons, the approach called MD Codes (see Figure 3.2.4) was developed to earn the ability of different injection guidelines, enabling the surgeon to be provided with precise location, delivery system, layer, tools and product quality and volume to achieve optimal results, as applied to the "great" collection of different faces. These results can be obtained regardless of ethnicity, age and gender differences.

Differences in technical skills and expertise of various surgeons may provide different outcomes, but MD Codes is a standardized way to achieve optimal results with a significant reduction in one's own manual variability, reducing the difference in resulting outcomes.

The MD Codes consist of a group of codes made up of numbers, letters, shapes and colors that represent defined and restricted anatomical areas on the face and also different applied procedures of HA filler injections, contouring and refilling, building up a language which can be known and applied by anyone in the world.

Any injection site is described using a combination of letters and numbers, where the letters mean anatomical units (e.g., chin, temple, cheek and so on) and the numbers mean subunits, i.e., each code indicates a single, defined, sharp injection site. For instance, the cheek is represented by the letters Ck, and subunits of the cheek are numbered as follows: Ck1 = zygomatic arch, Ck2 = zygomatic eminence, Ck3 = anteromedial cheek (mid-cheek) and so on.

MD Codes do not reflect any injection sequence but only a checklist of items, which can be marked once the surgeon approaches the facial aesthetics.

Those areas indicated in red are considered alarming zones (alert areas), including, for example, microcirculation of neuromuscular bundles [18]. Red codes can only be treated by highly trained and expert clinicians or surgeons—they must be cautious if using needles (cannulas are suggested) and pay particular attention throughout the whole process. While colors show dangerousness or hazards, shapes indicate how injections must be performed, i.e., injection delivery, e.g., bolus or linear injection.

Finally, each MD Code has also associated a target injection depth (e.g., supraperiosteal or subcutaneous), tolls (needle or cannula) and the minimal volume of HA filler (the active number). Needles are preferred for precise bolus injections upon the bone and/or when high precision and definition is requested, as occurring when treating fine lines in the subdermal plane (e.g., for lip lines). Cannulas are preferred for fat pad and subcutaneous injections or in the case where vessel bundles are in the proximity and may represent a concern.

BIBLIOGRAPHY

1. Rzany B, Cartier H, Kestermont P, Trevidic P, Sattler G, Kerrouche N, Dhuin JC. Correction of tear troughs and periorbital lines with a range of customized hyaluronic acid fillers. J Drugs Dermatol. 2012 Jan;11(1 Suppl):s27–34.
2. Rzany B, Cartier H, Kestemont P, Trevidic P, Sattler G, Kerrouche N, Dhuin JC, Ma YM. Full-face rejuvenation using a range of hyaluronic acid fillers: efficacy, safety, and patient satisfaction over 6 months. Dermatol Surg. 2012 Jul;38(7 Pt 2):1153–1161.
3. Ogilvie P, Safa M, Chantrey J, Leys C, Cavallini M, Niforos F, Hopfinger R, Marx A. Improvements in satisfaction with skin after treatment of facial fine lines with VYC-12 injectable gel: patient-reported outcomes from a prospective study. J Cosmet Dermatol. 2020 May;19(5):1065–1070.
4. Narurkar V, Shamban A, Sissins P, Stonehouse A, Gallagher C. Facial treatment preferences in aesthetically aware women. Dermatol Surg. 2015 Apr;41 Suppl 1:S153–S160.
5. Jagdeo J, Keaney T, Narurkar V, Kolodziejczyk J, Gallagher CJ. Facial treatment preferences among aesthetically oriented Men. Dermatol Surg. 2016 Oct;42(10):1155–1163.
6. Sobanko JF, Taglienti AJ, Wilson AJ, Sarwer DB, Margolis DJ, Dai J, Percec I. Motivations for seeking minimally invasive cosmetic procedures in an academic outpatient setting. Aesthet Surg J. 2015 Nov;35(8):1014–1020.
7. Sezgin B, Findikcioglu K, Kaya B, Sibar S, Yavuzer R. Mirror on the wall: a study of women's perception of facial features as they age. Aesthet Surg J. 2012 May;32(4):421–425.

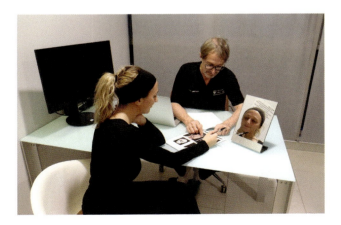

Figure 3.2.4 With a proper use of a scheme, we can explain to the patient a correct treatment plan.

8. Rubin MG, Cox SE, Kaminer MS, Solish N. Correcting age-related changes in the face by use of injectable fillers and neurotoxins. Semin Cutan Med Surg. 2014 Jun;33(4 Suppl):S81–S84.
9. Michaud T, Gassia V, Belhaouari L. Facial dynamics and emotional expressions in facial aging treatments. J Cosmet Dermatol. 2015 Mar;14(1):9–21.
10. Khan JA. Aesthetic surgery: diagnosing and healing the miscues of human facial expression. Ophthalmic Plast Reconstr Surg. 2001 Jan;17(1):4–6.
11. Charles Finn J, Cox SE, Earl ML. Social implications of hyperfunctional facial lines. Dermatol Surg. 2003 May;29(5):450–455.
12. Khan JA. Selective botulinum neurotoxin application: the interaction of evolution, biology, and culture in diagnosing and healing the miscues of human facial expression. Int Ophthalmol Clin. 2005 Summer;45(3):1–11.
13. Friedman O. Changes associated with the aging face. Facial Plast Surg Clin North Am. 2005 Aug;13(3):371–380.
14. Fitzgerald R. Contemporary concepts in brow and eyelid aging. Clin Plast Surg. 2013 Jan;40(1):21–42.
15. Knoll BI, Attkiss KJ, Persing JA. The influence of forehead, brow, and periorbital aesthetics on perceived expression in the youthful face. Plast Reconstr Surg. 2008 May;121(5):1793–1802.
16. De Maio M. Unlocking the code to facial revitalisation: a step-by-step approach to using injectables with the MD codesTM [pamphlet]. Dublin: Allergan Medical Institute; 2017.
17. De Maio M. Unlocking the messages of the face: addressing emotional attributes with the MD codesTM formulas [pamphlet]. Dublin: Allergan Medical Institute; 2017.
18. Scheuer JF 3rd, Sieber DA, Pezeshk RA, Campbell CF, Gassman AA, Rohrich RJ. Anatomy of the facial danger zones: maximizing safety during soft-tissue filler injections. Plast Reconstr Surg. 2017 Jan;139(1):50e–58e.

CHAPTER **4**

Preoperative Diagnostics

CHAPTER 4.1

Preoperative Diagnosis

Fernando Urdiales

INTRODUCTION

Treating patients with dermal fillers needs a thorough and continuous reassessment of practices to improve the ongoing and rapidly evolving aesthetic medicine and safeguard the patient's health. Crucial criteria are considered, including patient selection, filler knowledge and suboptimal injection approaches and techniques. To achieve this target, updated 10-point plans were forwarded in the field of non-surgical rhinoplasty and aesthetic medicine [1]. This plan is conceived to reduce the patient's involvement in undergoing complications associated with filler products or the surgeon's maneuvers and also to assess that the patient's health status does not promote any further side effects due to previous hampering conditions, such as skin pathologies (rosacea, dermatitis, acne), systemic or chronic diseases (hypersensitivity reactions such as allergy, autoimmunity, underlying viral diseases such as COVID-19 infection, herpes simplex, bacterial sepsis), medications (recreational drugs, chemopreventive therapies) and previous cosmetic treatments (energy-based treatments or fillers) [1]. The assessment of this wide panel of possible complications, to be completely prevented before any filler treatment, needs to update and make affordable, feasible and straightforward the current available devices and planning procedures to improve filler injections and aesthetic outcome, completely safeguarding patients' health.

An initial assessment should encompass the patient's needs, the role of social media and her or his relationship framework, including the patient's way of thinking about her or his life in the choice of aesthetic requests and a standardized photography. A thorough anamnestic interview should include a specific informed consent and information about previous adverse events, previous vascular or immune-inflammatory complications and previously performed aesthetic treatments. The surgeon or aesthetic physician must have a thorough knowledge of the filler product; the skill to select the best filler in the requested process; and follow a procedural step-by-step checklist encompassing consistent and reliable photograph documentation, a scheduled procedure plan, the inclusion of an aseptic non-touch technique, proper knowledge of topographical anatomy of the injectable region and its boundaries, knowledge of possible angiosome existence, technical dexterity in pinch anatomy and skill in injection practice, all points of paramount importance. Preinjection aspiration of the hyaluronic acid (HA) filler is a controversial technique, recently reviewed in its impact in aesthetic medicine [4].

Preventing complications around the dermal filler-related procedures requires the use of technical practices and devices to better diagnose pretreatment issues leading to possible adverse events, devices which usually are more commonly considered for surgical interventions, but which are being considered more and more in dermal filler application and in non-surgical rhinoplasty. Improving the use of imaging technologies to better focus on anatomical and physio-pathological items able to affect the outcome of a dermal filler is of paramount interest for the best practice in the field.

MAGNETIC RESONANCE IMAGING (MRI)

A modest bulk of publications dealing with MRI in dermal fillers exist in the scientific literature so far [5–11]. Though increasing in interest and numbers, these reports are still poorly acknowledged in describing filler behavior in an MRI context to prevent further filler-associated complications. From a biochemical point of view, HA is a glycosaminoglycan and rapidly biodegradable, which is naturally present in the extracellular matrix of dermal tissue, having a role in maintaining both structure and functional integrity of the skin. The hydrophilic features of HA allow the molecule to attract water, maintaining hydration in the filler-injected areas, i.e., wherever HA fillers are injected or natural HA is present [12]. HA acid fillers, known as medium-term fillers, are usually designed to last from three months to one year [8]. Therefore, the HA signal in MRI closely follows the water MRI signal due to HA biochemical composition and the hydrophilic features [13]. Furthermore, filler presence can be easily identified and separated from fats and other tissues. The cross-sectional MRI allows the user to identify further structures such as the surface musculoaponeurotic system, which is particularly crucial for the physician to identify [14].

Some authors have recommended an MRI protocol (in sequence) for the face imaging as follows: a) 3 mm for sagittal T2 (weighted for fat saturation) and sagittal T1; b) 2 mm for axial T2 (weighted for fat saturation) and axial T1; c) 4 mm for axial diffusion; d) 3 mm for coronal T2 (weighted for fat saturation); and e) 3 mm for post-contrast sagittal T1 [15]. The anatomical localization of the HA filler with MRI is particularly easy to achieve. Taking into consideration the possible complications related to HA fillers, the buttocks are probably the most frequently affected area [16].

On the face, complications often involve the periocular region, perioral area, malar fat pad, nasolabial folds, glabella, marionette lines and lips [17] (see Figures 4.1.1 and 4.1.2). Moreover, diffuse patterns have been reported in the periorbital and the nasal pyramid regions, but also infiltration into the lips [16]. MRI has allowed the ability to detect non-inflammatory nodules, abscesses and granulomas, where the imaging technique results were helpful to achieve a differential diagnosis, particularly when the depth of complications involves the muscle underneath [17,18]. Whereas with computed tomography (CT), the soft tissue attenuation is considered a common sign of the presence of HA fillers (see Figure 4.1.3), in MRI, HA fillers show a substantial hyperintense signal

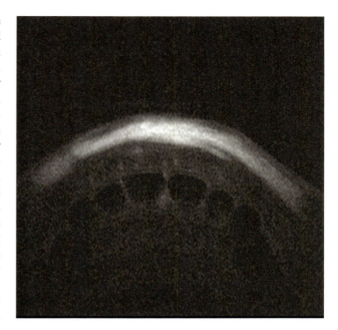

Figure 4.1.1 MRI image showing the filler distribution into the muscle.

on T2 and short tau inversion recovery (STIR) sequences, whereas a hypointense signal is on T1 weighted sequences because of the high content in water [16]. Usually, following the first six months postinjection, a minor postcontrast enhancement can be viewed, probably due to an enhancement in vascularization within the interested area [16].

MRI is able to detect facial complications due to biased HA filler procedures. In the case of abscess formation, it is

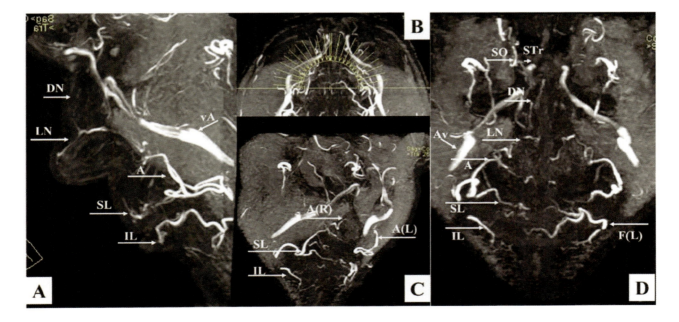

Figure 4.1.2 MRI image showing the facial vascularization.

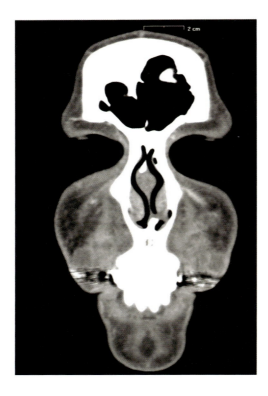

Figure 4.1.3 TC scan showing the HA filler into the soft tissues.

formula. Low-viscosity SO is somehow hyperintense with respect to water on T1 weighted MRI, isointense or moderately ipointense on T2 weighted, as well as high-viscous SO, whereas on CT, it is slightly hyperintense [16–20].

ULTRASOUND TECHNIQUES

Ultrasound-guided diagnosis (UGD) is a novel technique to diagnose filler-associated complications and drive a possible therapy intervention (see Figure 4.1.4). The device, which usually consists of a probe and a processor, by generating ultrasound waves is able to penetrate tissues and interacting with the same are absorbed, buffered or scattered, thus providing different reflected sound waves (echoes) that are turned into electronic signals and finally into an imaging output by the processor. Different echogenicity reflects the presence or absence of a particular substance, such as the HA filler. UGD terminology is particularly easy to learn. No echoes result in a black image on UGD (anechoic), various shades of dark gray mean low amounts of echoes (hypoechoic), echo-rich zones—various shades of light-gray—are hyperechoic with respect to neighboring structures, whereas UGD areas with similar echogenicity of adjoining structures are isoechoic [21]. Furthermore, it is possible to integrate a Doppler system with a UGD, forming a duplex device [21]. Duplex can highlight microcirculation as red and blue colors, to be identified in relation with other structures. As HA fillers are hydrophilic compounds, their UGD signal depends on the HA relationship with the surrounding tissue echogenicity. Water does not reflect ultrasound waves, and therefore HA fillers are usually non-echogenic (non-echoic) or hypoechoic.

possible that the natural barrier of the skin is interrupted by using HA filler injection, thus enhancing the further possibility of infections. Migration of fillers or overfilling can also occur, mimicking a malignant pathology if colonizing lymph nodes and appears in MRI as a diffuse facial asymmetry or as focal lumps.

In MRI, the abscess usually shows a restricted diffusion on diffusion weighted imaging (DWI), as it appears as a lobulated fluid accumulation with a clear enhancement of the adjacent fat stranding on MRI and the rim [19]. Foreign body granulomas and non-inflammatory nodules are rarely seen with HA fillers but usually with silicone oil (SO) infusion, which has characteristic features in MRI, depending on its viscosity or purified

Vascular complications due to HA filler injections can be easily detected with a Doppler UGD [22] (DUS), and usually UGD is easier and more feasible than MRI, which is ultimately used for surgical decision making [23]. DUS is a formidable tool to an anatomically guided HA filler injection procedure in order to minimize drastically any

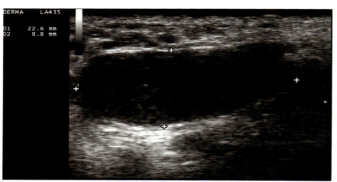 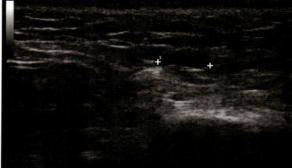

Figure 4.1.4 Ultrasound showing a deposit of filler into the soft tissues.

complication associated with the dermal filler [24]. UGD is therefore a non-invasive technique able to visualize HA fillers and possible dermis modifications due to fillers or skin bioptic withdrawals [25]. From this perspective, any dermal change over a long-term period is monitored by UGD, because cysts, granulomas or other skin lesions and pathologies may occur with HA filler treatment. When Juvederm Voluma is used, a kind of serpiginous deposition may be formed, locally quite sharp but with shallow delineation, resulting in a partially heterogeneous imaging from hypoechogenous to clearly hyperechogenous, depending on the practical procedure employed [26].

ENDOSCOPIC DIAGNOSIS AND INSTRUMENTATION TOOLS

Endoscopic sinus surgery is one field of application in continuous expansion and finds the reasons for its development thanks to the achievements of technology [27,28]. The operator must have acquired a technical knowledge of the relative surgical instruments and the intrinsic characteristics of the endoscope itself (dimensions, viewing angle, etc.) along with its numerous accessories (light source, camera, monitor, video recording system, etc.). Adequate tools are the key to improving the quality of the surgical act by significantly reducing operating times [29]. The optics are the starting tools for any endoscopy and therefore also for endoscopic surgery. The rigid endoscope has changed considerably over time since it was introduced by Hopkins in England. Industries at the forefront of their marketing are currently Storz and Wolf [30]. The endoscope is illuminated by a cold light produced by a light source (halogen or xenon) by means of a fiber optic cable.

There are different sizes (from 2.7 to 4 mm in diameter) and different viewing angles (from 0 to 120 degrees) with a depth of focus from 10 to 80 mm. There is a standard and wide-angle version of each instrument. Optics of sufficient diameter are usually used to allow a good visualization of the surgical field. Therefore, the 4 mm optic is the most frequently used. How many at the viewing angle, the most commonly used endoscopes are 0, 30 and 70 degrees.

A 0-degree optic (direct forward vision) 4 mm is the main tool for any endoscopic sinus surgery. Most of the surgical maneuvers are performed under the visual control of this endoscope. Due to the forward orientation of the visual field, it is the only endoscope whose major axis always points directly into the direction of the gaze (i.e., directly along the axis of the shaft), so it is the tool of choice for newbies.

The 4-mm endoscope also allows a forward view at an angle of 30 degrees. It is a highly diagnostic tool because it allows you to explore, thanks to the orientation of its distal lens, the middle meatus, the maxillary sinus through the natural ostium, the sphenoethmoidal recess and the nasopharynx. The advantage is that it often allows the surgeon to perform the entire surgery without having to change optics.

The 4-mm 70-degree endoscope is used in some particular surgical situations within the maxillary sinus or on the frontal recess. Not allowing the view along the shaft of the instrument requires considerable attention and experience to avoid contact with the mucosa and consequent injuries during its introduction.

The 120-degree endoscope is the exclusive prerogative of the maxillary sinus, for example, for inspecting the anterior wall of the sinus. Other optics with intermediate angles—25 and 45 degrees—are used in particular situations to better dominate the "hidden corners" of the surgical field.

The sinuscopy trocar with oblique tip is used to introduce the optics described earlier if a sinuscopy is performed through the canine fossa.

Endoscopic surgery is a procedure that is performed mainly with one hand by connecting the endoscope to an external display system. For the neophyte, it can be difficult to dissociate the manual act of the visualization axis and the degree of optical distortion that makes depth perception difficult. These potential difficulties are more than compensated for by the remarkable clarity of the endoscopic image, by the ability to move the instrument freely within the nasal cavity and by an excellent "spatial sensation" thanks to the surgeon's ability to see beyond the corners. It also obviously has the advantages of collegial vision with the possible use of a registration system.

Finally, it is useful to remember that the appropriate visualization of the operating field also depends on the cleaning of the end portion of the optics—simple irrigation of the operating field with lukewarm saline and subsequently frequent aspiration help obtain a good view of the surgical field.

OTHER TECHNIQUES

The level of placement of HA fillers may depend extensively on the various indications intended to be addressed and by the facial anatomy of the targeted area, as well as the HA filler product, biochemical composition formulas and further approved indications. Injectable cosmetic fillers can possess a radiolucency/soft tissue density in CT and cone beam CT (CBCT), including HA, collagen and fat. Radiopaque fillers can be described on plain radiographs, such as panoramic radiographs, yet are surely better detailed in CT and CBCT, as reported by many experts in the field [31–36].

CONCLUSIONS

Using the best prediagnostic devices, tools and methods in the management of dermal fillers is of paramount interest. The proper choice of prediagnostic tools depends on technique affordability, feasibility and straightforward applicability in order to obtain rigorous data about the patient's situation and engage in the best planned procedure to achieve the optimal result with less time-consuming bias, less turn-around time for procedures and the best aesthetic results for patients' health and satisfaction.

BIBLIOGRAPHY

1. Heydenrych I, De Boulle K, Kapoor KM, Bertossi D. The 10-point plan 2021: updated concepts for improved procedural safety during facial filler treatments. Clin Cosmet Investig Dermatol. 2021 Jul 6;14:779–814.
2. Heydenrych I, Kapoor KM, De Boulle K, Goodman G, Swift A, Kumar N, Rahman E. A 10-point plan for avoiding hyaluronic acid dermal filler-related complications during facial aesthetic procedures and algorithms for management. Clin Cosmet Investig Dermatol. 2018 Nov 23;11:603–611.
3. Urdiales-Gálvez F, Delgado NE, Figueiredo V, Lajo-Plaza JV, Mira M, Ortíz-Martí F, Del Rio-Reyes R, Romero-Álvarez N, Del Cueto SR, Segurado MA, Rebenaque CV. Preventing the complications associated with the use of dermal fillers in facial aesthetic procedures: an expert group consensus report. Aesthetic Plast Surg. 2017 Jun;41(3):667–677.
4. Kapoor KM, Murthy R, Hart SLA, Cattin TA, Nola PF, Rossiter AP, Singh R, Singh S. Factors influencing pre-injection aspiration for hyaluronic acid fillers: a systematic literature review and meta-analysis. Dermatol Ther. 2021 Jan;34(1):e14360.
5. Jeong KH, Gwak MJ, Moon SK, Lee SJ, Shin MK. Efficacy and durability of hyaluronic acid fillers for malar enhancement: a prospective, randomized, split-face clinical controlled trial. J Cosmet Laser Ther. 2018 Jun;20(3):184–188.
6. Kadouch JA, Tutein Nolthenius CJ, Kadouch DJ, van der Woude HJ, Karim RB, Hoekzema R. Complications after facial injections with permanent fillers: important limitations and considerations of MRI evaluation. Aesthet Surg J. 2014 Aug;34(6):913–923.
7. Di Girolamo M, Mattei M, Signore A, Grippaudo FR. MRI in the evaluation of facial dermal fillers in normal and complicated cases. Eur Radiol. 2015 May;25(5):1431–1442.
8. Tal S, Maresky HS, Bryan T, Ziv E, Klein D, Persitz A, Heller L. MRI in detecting facial cosmetic injectable fillers. Head Face Med. 2016 Sep 6;12(1):27.
9. Kadouch JA, Tutein Nolthenius CJ, Kadouch DJ, van der Woude HJ, Karim RB, Hoekzema R. Complications after facial injections with permanent fillers: important limitations and considerations of MRI evaluation. Aesthet Surg J. 2014 Aug;34(6):913–923.
10. Costa ALF, Caliento R, da Rocha GBL, Gomes JPP, Mansmith AJC, de Freitas CF, Braz-Silva PH. Magnetic resonance imaging appearance of foreign-body granulomatous reactions to dermal cosmetic fillers. Imaging Sci Dent. 2017 Dec;47(4):281–284.
11. Mespreuve M, Waked K, Collard B, De Ranter J, Vanneste F, Hendrickx B. The usefulness of magnetic resonance angiography to analyze the variable arterial facial anatomy in an effort to reduce filler-associated blindness: anatomical study and visualization through an augmented reality application. Aesthet Surg J Open Forum. 2021 May 11;3(3):ojab018.
12. Beasley KL, Weiss MA, Weiss RA. Hyaluronic acid fillers: a comprehensive review. Facial Plast Surg. 2009 May;25(2):86–94.
13. Murthy R, Roos JCP, Goldberg RA. Periocular hyaluronic acid fillers: applications, implications, complications. Curr Opin Ophthalmol. 2019 Sep;30(5):395–400.
14. Cotofana S, Fratila AA, Schenck TL, Redka-Swoboda W, Zilinsky I, Pavicic T. The anatomy of the aging face: a review. Facial Plast Surg. 2016 Jun;32(3):253–260.
15. Master M. Hyaluronic acid filler longevity and localization: magnetic resonance imaging evidence. Plast Reconstr Surg. 2021 Jan 1;147(1):50e–53e.
16. Gonzalez-Hermosillo LM, Ramos-Pacheco VH, Gonzalez-Hermosillo DC, Cervantes-Sanchez AM, Vega-Gutierrez AE, Ternovoy SK, Roldan-Valadez E. MRI visualization and distribution patterns of foreign modeling agents: a brief pictorial review for clinicians. Biomed Res Int. 2021 Nov 29;2021:2838246.
17. Mundada P, Kohler R, Boudabbous S, Toutous Trellu L, Platon A, Becker M. Injectable facial fillers: imaging features, complications, and diagnostic pitfalls at MRI and PET CT. Insights Imaging. 2017 Dec;8(6):557–572.
18. Martínez-Villarreal AA, Asz-Sigall D, Gutiérrez-Mendoza D, Serena TE, Lozano-Platonoff A, Sanchez-Cruz LY, Toussaint-Caire S, Domínguez-Cherit J, López-García LA, Cárdenas-Sánchez A, Contreras-Ruiz J. A case series and a review of the literature on foreign modelling agent reaction: an emerging problem. Int Wound J. 2017 Jun;14(3):546–554.
19. Harish S, Chiavaras MM, Kotnis N, Rebello R. MR imaging of skeletal soft tissue infection: utility of diffusion-weighted imaging in detecting abscess formation. Skeletal Radiol. 2011 Mar;40(3):285–294.
20. Ginat DT, Schatz CJ. Imaging of facial fillers: additional insights. AJNR Am J Neuroradiol. 2012 Dec;33(11):E140–E141.
21. Schelke LW, Decates TS, Velthuis PJ. Ultrasound to improve the safety of hyaluronic acid filler treatments. J Cosmet Dermatol. 2018 Dec;17(6):1019–1024.
22. Lee AL, Chen YF, Yao WT, Liu YC, Yu CM, Yu CM, Tu CP, Huang WC, Tung KY, Tsai MF. Laser doppler imaging for treating vascular complications from procedures involving dermal fillers: case series and literature review. Diagnostics (Basel). 2021 Sep 7;11(9):1640.
23. Carella S, Ruggeri G, La Russa R, Volonnino G, Frati P, Onesti MG. Clinical management of complications following filler injection. Aesthetic Plast Surg. 2021 Nov 23. doi: 10.1007/s00266-021-02650-4.

24. Velthuis PJ, Jansen O, Schelke LW, Moon HJ, Kadouch J, Ascher B, Cotofana S. A guide to doppler ultrasound analysis of the face in cosmetic medicine. Part 1: standard positions. Aesthet Surg J. 2021 Oct 15;41(11):NP1621–NP1632.
25. Qiao J, Jia QN, Jin HZ, Li F, He CX, Yang J, Zuo YG, Fu LQ. Long-term follow-up of longevity and diffusion pattern of hyaluronic acid in nasolabial fold correction through high-frequency ultrasound. Plast Reconstr Surg. 2019 Aug;144(2):189e–196e.
26. Vandeputte J, Leemans G, Dhaene K, Forsyth R, Vanslembrouck J, Hatem F, Micheels P. Spreading pattern and tissue response to hyaluronic acid gel injections in the subcutis: ultrasound videos, ultrasound measurements, and histology. Aesthet Surg J. 2021 Jan 25;41(2):224–241.
27. Kennedy DW, Senior BA. Endoscopic sinus surgery: a review. Otolariyngol Clin North Am. 1997 Jun;30(3):313–330.
28. Hosemann WG, Weber RK, Keerl RE, Lund VJ. Minimally invasive endonasal sinus surgery. Thieme; 2000, pp. 106–107.
29. Modugno CG, Sciarretta V, Pasquini E. Il contributo della tecnologia nella chirurgia endoscopica. XLVII Raduno Gruppo Oto-Rino_Laringologico Alta Italia, 22–23.
30. Wigand ME, Hoseman W. Endoscopic surgery of the paranasal sinuses and anterior skull base. Thieme; 1990.
31. Alsufyani NA, Alsufyani MA. Radiographic features of facial cosmetic material: report of two cases. Case Rep Dent. 2021 Sep 30;2021:7308636.
32. Cabrera MA, Mulinari-Brenner F. Radiological evaluation of calcium hydroxyapatite-based cutaneous fillers. Surgical and Cosmetic Dermatology. 2011;3(3):203–205.
33. Koka S, Shah K, Mallya S. Dermal filler presenting as lobular radiopacities in an edentulous patient: a clinical report. Journal of Prosthodontics. 2017;26(8):670–671.
34. Kwon Y, An C, Choi KS, Lee D, An S. Radiographic study of dermal fillers in the facial area: a series of 3 cases. Imaging Science in Dentistry. 2018;48(3):227–231.
35. Mundada P, Kohler R, Boudabbous S, Toutous Trellu L, Platon A, Becker M. Injectable facial fillers: imaging features, complications, and diagnostic pitfalls at MRI and PET CT. Insights into Imaging. 2017;8(6):557–572.
36. Valiyaparambil JR, Rengasamy K, Mallya SM. An unusual soft tissue radiopacity: Radiographic appearance of a dermal filler. British Dental Journal. 2009;207(5):211–212.

CHAPTER 4.2

Skin Conditions Affecting the Nose and Perinasal Area

Izolda Heydenrych

INTRODUCTION

The nose, by virtue of its centrofacial location, constitutes a focal point of interest to both the patient and injector. As such, overt skin pathology has often been addressed before the request for non-surgical rhinoplasty. There are, however, countless subtle and undiagnosed conditions that may have direct bearing on both injection safety and outcomes.

Importantly, the nose is supremely exposed not only to sight but also to the exposome, predisposing to the formation of both precancerous and cancerous lesions, which may necessitate cosmetically undesirable surgery if diagnosed late. In addition, the nasal skin is prone to numerous inflammatory and infective conditions which serve as a relative contraindication to the safe treatment with fillers. Conditions such as acne, dermatitis and herpes simplex mandate adequate pretreatment despite possible subtle presentations. It is the prerogative of the careful injector to recognize these conditions and the need for treatment and to plan the timing of filler injections accordingly (Table 4.2.1) [1].

The desired prerequisites for healthy skin prior to surgical rhinoplasty have been summarized as [2]:

- Even texture (keratinocyte exfoliation)
- Even color (melanocyte production and distribution)
- Optimal hydration
- Disease-free (melasma, rosacea, etc.)
- Tolerant (good barrier function)
- Normal contour
- Firm/tight (fibroblast production of collagen and elastin)

The important prerequisite for non-surgical rhinoplasty is disease-free skin with good barrier function, as this is particularly important in avoiding late-onset adverse events. Accurate diagnosis and pretreatment of conditions commonly affecting the nose are thus vital, mandating accurate diagnosis and knowledge of current treatment options. It is also vital that procedures are planned to allow adequate restoration of barrier function, which may take up to one month after apparent clearing in conditions such as dermatitis [1,3].

CONDITIONS MANDATING PRETREATMENT BEFORE FILLER PROCEDURES

Before non-surgical rhinoplasty, disease-free skin with good barrier function is particularly important in order to avoid immune stimulation, infection and development of late-onset adverse events (LOAEs).

INFECTIVE/INFLAMMATORY CONDITIONS

Skin barrier disruption, which may be due to either infective or inflammatory conditions, predisposes to penetration of infective agents, thus posing a risk factor for LOAEs.

After skin penetration, pathogens bind to the NOD-like and toll-like receptors (TLRs) to induce an immune stimulus which may lead to the formation of LOAEs up to a year later. It is thus vitally important that conditions such as acne, rosacea, perioral dermatitis and seborrheic dermatitis are fully pretreated and that the filler procedure is scheduled after full recovery of barrier function.

Importantly, LOAEs may also ensue after hematogenous spread of underlying systemic infections, which should be carefully excluded during consultation. A detailed history of current medications should be sought in order to elucidate underlying conditions such as urinary tract infections, sinusitis, gastroenteritis or dental caries.

For planning purposes, the importance of a prefiller consultation cannot be overemphasized, with varying optimal procedural timings, as indicated in the existing literature [3].

SKIN CONDITIONS AFFECTING THE NOSE AND PERINASAL AREA

Table 4.2.1 Conditions Requiring Pretreatment Before Fillers and Suggested Timings

Condition	Contraindication (CI) or Physician Discretion (PD)	Timing to Filler	Suggestions
Acne	CI/PD	Clearance	Topical: Pretreat entire acne area ↑ Resistant *Cutibacterium acnes* at edge of topically treated area; no safe distance
Rosacea	CI/PD	Control +/− 12 weeks	Barrier restoration is vital.
Perioral dermatitis	CI/PD	6 weeks	Eliminate causes, e.g., steroids (topical, inhalant)
Dermatitis	CI/PD	3-4 weeks after apparent clearance	Caution: allergies, *Staphylococcus* carriers, eczema herpeticum
Herpes simplex	CI	Infective until last crusts disappeared	Prophylaxis if history
Previous late-onset adverse event	PD	1 month after full clearance	Elucidate and avoid predisposing factors Dermal test if allergic
Impetigo	CI	Total clearance	Treat carrier status

HERPES SIMPLEX VIRUS

Etiopathogenesis: Herpes simplex virus (HSV) types 1 and 2 cause a ubiquitous condition establishing lifelong infections in humans. Although the major transmission route for HSV-1 is oral and type HSV-2 is sexual, lesion location is not necessarily indicative of the viral type and may vary among unique subpopulations. Infection is often latent and asymptomatic, with frequent reactivations, which may manifest after perioral needle stick injury from fillers. Intermittent symptomatic episodes are common [4]. Importantly, occult lesions may also occur in the nares. HSV lesions are infective until disappearance of the last crust.

In patients with a history of HSV, the condition is best treated prophylactically starting one day pretreatment and for the full five days in order to avoid the development of eczema herpeticum in needle prick areas. This is important especially when injecting close to HSV areas and in those with a history of active atopic dermatitis [3] (see Figure 4.2.1).

Prophylactic treatment: Acyclovir, valacyclovir, famciclovir, starting one day prefiller for five days.

Filler timing: Lesions are infective until disappearance of last crusts.

Risks: Eczema herpeticum.

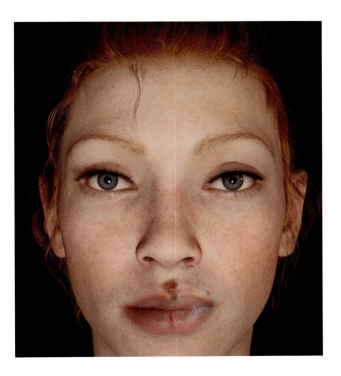

Figure 4.2.1 Patient demonstrating HSV of the upper lip and left nares. Importantly, lesions are infective until disappearance of the last crusts. It is advisable to treat these lesions up-front before fillers or lasers in order to avoid koebnerization. Treatment was with oral valacyclovir 500 mg bd × 5 days.

IMPETIGO

Etiopathogenesis: Impetigo is a highly contagious bacterial skin infection caused by *Staphylococcus aureus* or *Streptococcus pyogenes*. It presents clinically in either non-bullous (70%) or bullous form. The non-bullous form is characterized by the presence of small pustules which quickly develop yellowish-brown crusted plaques. The presentation may be insidious in adults. Bullous impetigo is caused by *S. aureus* and usually presents as large bullae.

The incidence of asymptomatic and permanent *S. aureus* nasal colonization is cited as up to 30%, which may lead to opportunistic and sometimes life-threatening infections after both surgical and non-surgical procedures. This increases morbidity, mortality and healthcare costs. Importantly, *S. aureus* may be transmitted from healthcare workers, with mobile phones proven to be a potential reservoir. Smokers are more frequently colonized than non-smokers, with cessation from smoking having been shown to improve clearance.

The presence of *S. aureus* in the nares induces both innate and adaptive immune systems in order to overcome the bacteria. When host defense mechanisms are suboptimal, it may also predispose to chronic furunculosis, as seen in atopic patients [5].

Treatment: Topical mupirocin is currently the first-line therapy, with retapamulin and fusidic acid posing alternative options. Patients with numerous lesions or unresponsive to topical treatment may be treated with an oral antibiotic, with options including dicloxacillin, amoxicillin/clavulanate and cephalexin. Microbial culture with sensitivity is advisable in these patients [6].

Carrier status may be treated with intranasal mupirocin 2% thrice daily for 6 days [7].

ACNE

Etiopathogenesis: Acne vulgaris is a common, multifactorial inflammatory disease of the pilosebaceous follicles affecting approximately 10% of individuals worldwide [8]. It is characterized by open or closed comedones and inflammatory lesions (papules, pustules, nodules or cysts).

Key pathogenic factors include follicular hyperkeratinization, microbial colonization with *Cutibacterium acnes* (which are present in all acne lesions, whether comedonal or inflammatory), excess sebum production and complex inflammatory mechanisms involving both innate and acquired immunity. Neuroendocrine regulation, diet and genetic factors may also play a role [9] (see Figure 4.2.2).

Importantly, *C. acnes* may cause opportunistic infections and biofilms when their physiological niche is disturbed by medical device–related trauma such as filler treatments [8]. There is no documented "safe area" for injection relative to acne in other facial areas, and these should be adequately treated before non-surgical rhinoplasty (see Figure x). Also, patients tend to pick at their skins potentially transferring acne pathogens (see Figure 4.2.3).

Treatment: Topical therapies include benzoyl peroxide (BP) and topical retinoids, with combination adapalene 0.1%/BP 2.5% being the first-line therapy. Topical treatment with fixed-dose combination BP/adapalene gel leads to a 29% reduction in lesion count after 12 weeks of treatment [10]. Systemic medications include doxycycline, lymecycline, hormonal agents and isotretinoin [9].

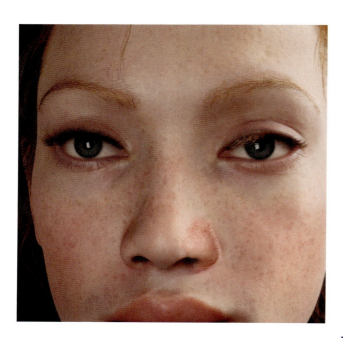

Figure 4.2.2 Patient demonstrating comedonal acne of the nasal area. Although non-inflammatory, comedones harbor *Cutibacterium acnes*, which may predispose to biofilms and LOAEs should their physiological niche be disturbed. This patient should be pretreated with topical acne medication before fillers.

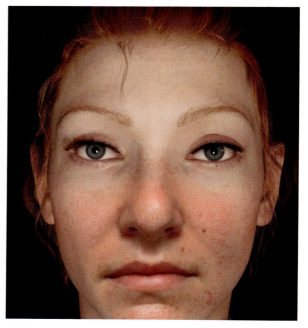

Figure 4.2.3 Patient demonstrating inflammatory acne of the lower face and underlying rosacea. Note the non-inflammatory comedones in addition to inflammatory papules, pustules and scarring. There is no documented "safe area" for adjacent filler treatment. This patient with resistant, scarring acne was treated with isotretinoin 0.5 mg/kg/day to a total dose of 120 mg/kg.

ROSACEA

Etiopathogenesis: Rosacea is a common, chronic, inflammatory facial dermatosis with a multivariate disease process underlying various clinical manifestations. The pathogenesis is an inflammatory continuum, including alterations in the innate system, neurovascular dysregulation, cutaneous microflora (demodex folliculorum, bacillus oleranius) and inflammatory mediators such as cathelicidin, antimicrobial peptides, defensins and alarmins. Of great practical importance is the disruption of the skin barrier system, which may be equal to that found in atopic dermatitis (see Figures 4.2.4 and 4.2.5).

Clinical manifestations: Erythemato-telangiectatic, papulopustular and phymatous variants were previously described, with more than 50% of patients also manifesting ocular changes. A new classification is based on morphological features.

Treatment: Combination treatments to target subtype and clinical features, appropriate skincare and lifestyle modifications (avoidance of trigger factors such as heat, cold, spicy foods, alcohol, emotional stress).

Topical: Ivermectin 1% cream, metronidazole gel 1%, azelaic acid 15%, topical minocycline foam.

Systemic: Doxycycline, lymecycline, low-dose isotretinoin.

Energy-based devices: For vascular dilatation and persistent erythema: pulsed dye laser, potassium titanyl phosphate (KTP) laser and intense pulsed light (IPL) therapy.

Isotretinoin is indicated for the treatment of acne, rosacea, rhinophyma and sebaceous hyperplasia. It may also be used presurgically to treat aesthetically undesirable thick skin, complementing rhinoplasty by controlling sebum production and uniformly thinning the skin-subcutaneous tissue envelope without compromising the underlying bony and cartilaginous nasal structures. Isotretinoin may also serve to prevent posttreatment acne flares, thus embodying an invaluable tool in the skin's treatment armamentarium [12].

The optimal dosage varies according to indication. Nodulocystic or resistant acne may require a dose of 0.5–1 mg/kg to a total cumulative dose of 120 mg/kg. It should be kept in mind that higher doses may cause both dryness and skin fragility while on treatment, which should be managed proactively. Rosacea dosages are generally lower, ranging between 10 and 20 mg/day for three months [13]. Due to the inherent dry skin and barrier deficiency associated with erythemato-telangiectatic rosacea (ETR), optimal moisturization, preferably with ceramide-containing moisturizes, is vital [14]. In rosacea patients, particular care should be exercised in avoiding ocular dryness and the risk of corneal ulceration. The dosage and duration for refining nasal skin vary. The suggested dosage is 10–20 mg/kg for three months.

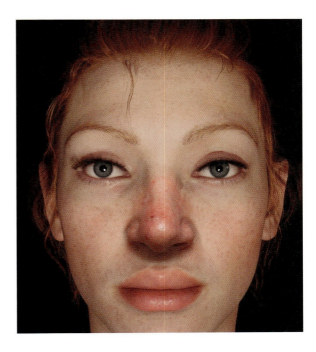

Figure 4.2.4 Patient demonstrating pustular rosacea of the nose. Pretreatment of the rosacea, with stabilization of barrier function and reduction in demodex folliculorum, is advised in these patients. Treatment was with topical 1% ivermectin cream and oral lymecycline (300 mg/day) for three months.

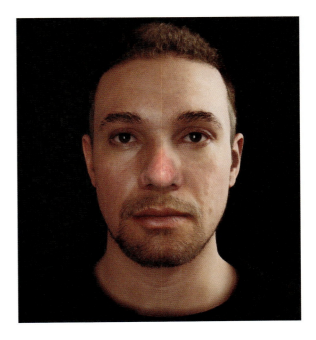

Figure 4.2.5 Patient with erythemato-telangiectatic rosacea (ETR), telangiectasia and fibrous changes of the nasal skin. Importantly ETR demonstrates profound changes in barrier function and loss of hydration similar to that found in atopic dermatitis [11]. Treatment was with isotretinoin 10 mg/day, and the telangiectasia was addressed with pulsed dye laser. Note the small fibrous papule in the left paranasal region.

Table 4.2.2 Acne and Rosacea Characterization

	Acne Vulgaris	Rosacea
Chronic inflammatory disease	+	+
Centrofacial flushing	− Perilesional erythema may be present	+ Flushing may be more imperceptible in darker skin types
Comedones	+	−
Papules + pustules	+/−	+/−
Areas affected	Widespread, also lateral face	Centrofacial
Occurrence	Chronic	Episodic
Triggers	Various	Sun, heat, alcohol, emotions, spicy foods, hot beverages
Ocular involvement	−	+ (>50%)
Skin barrier dysfunction	−	+++
Postinflammatory hyperpigmentation	More common	Less common

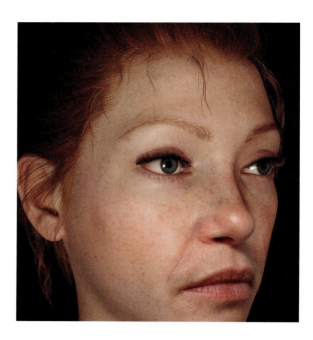

Figure 4.2.6 Perioral dermatitis manifests as small papules and scant pustules in the perioral and paranasal region. There was a history of topical steroid creams for what was considered underlying dermatitis. This patient was treated with lymecycline 300 mg/day for six weeks and strict avoidance of topical steroids.

PERIORAL DERMATITIS

Etiopathogenesis: Perioral dermatitis (POD) is a cutaneous eruption affecting the perioral, perinasal and sometimes periocular areas. It occurs most commonly in women and children and is characterized by an acneiform eruption, often with an additional eczematous appearance. Classically there is a ring of uninvolved skin adjacent to the vermillion border of the lips. Both classical and granulomatous subtypes are described. The features often resemble those of rosacea, both clinically and histologically. Patients require an evaluation of etiologic factors, the most important of which is the use of topical or even inhaled steroids.

Treatment options include avoidance of steroids, oral and skin rinses after steroid inhalants, oral tetracyclines (six weeks), topical metronidazole, topical azelaic acid, adapalene gel, pimecrolimus cream and oral isotretinoin [15]. For underlying dermatitis in patients prone to perioral dermatitis or patients with rosacea, topical calcineurin inhibitors such as pimecrolimus cream are a good alternative (see Figure 4.2.6).

DERMATITIS

Etiopathogenesis: Patients may present with the request for fillers while demonstrating various types and degrees of dermatitis, including seborrheic, contact and irritant dermatitis.

Whereas seborrheic dermatitis commonly affects the paranasal region, contact dermatitis does not commonly affect the dorsal or alar regions. This is consistent with studies citing average skin thickness as an important parameter for allergen/irritant penetration, with the thickest dermis occurring in the lower nasal sidewall [16].

Although facial dermatitis (FD) in women is well characterized, recent trends in the male grooming industry have implicated unique sources of allergens for male facial contact dermatitis, with referrals for patch testing in males doubling over the past two decades. Allergic rhinitis has been shown to be associated with FD in all genders [17].

A history of, and reasons for, contact and irritant dermatitis should be carefully elucidated, as the propensity may also have a bearing on preprocedural cleansers and postprocedural topicals. Importantly, skin barrier function may take three to four weeks after apparent clearing of dermatitis to return to normal (see Figure 4.2.7).

SEBORRHEIC DERMATITIS

Etiopathogenesis: Seborrheic dermatitis (SD) is a common, relapsing inflammatory skin disease occurring more often in males. The prevalence is lower during the summer months, possibly due to ultraviolet (UV)-induced immunosuppressive effects on the cutaneous microbiome [19].

Although the morphology may be heterogeneous, SD characteristically occurs in sebaceous areas (paranasal, eyebrows, hairline, postauricular, scalp) as poorly demarcated erythematous patches with accompanying greasy scaling [19].

SKIN CONDITIONS AFFECTING THE NOSE AND PERINASAL AREA

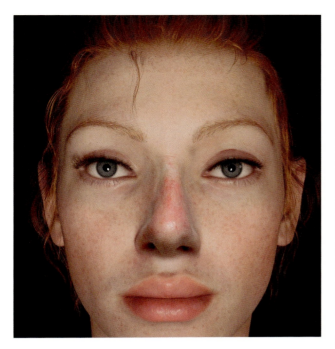

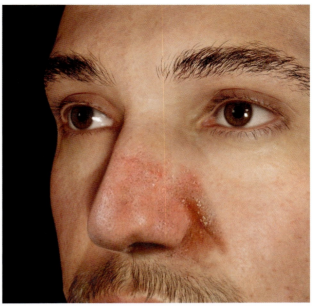

Figure 4.2.8 Seborrheic dermatitis of the paranasal groove and medial cheek (18). Note the greasy, yellow scale.

Figure 4.2.7 Patient demonstrating irritant dermatitis with excoriations on the dorsal nose. Suboptimal barrier function is common in these patients [18]. This patient was treated with bland emollients and daily topical 0.1% methylprednisolone aceponate (a non-atrophogenic steroid) for one week, weaned over one month. Avoidance of the causative irritant is mandatory. Note the inflammatory erythema.

Both host and environmental factors are cited as pathogenetic determinants. Overgrowth of commensal *Malassezia* species in a predisposed host is implicated, with several studies underlining the pathogenetic importance of decreased skin barrier function in SD [20].

Treatment includes general skincare with soap substitutes and appropriate moisturizers. Interventions aimed at improving skin barrier function are increasingly mentioned. Medical treatment includes topical antifungals, mild topical steroids and topical calcineurin inhibitors.

In severe, generalized disease or refractory cases, oral treatment with itraconazole, ketoconazole or low-dose isotretinoin may be attempted [21]. **Non-malignant neoplastic conditions**

SEBACEOUS HYPERPLASIA

Etiopathogenesis: Sebaceous hyperplasia (SH) is the most common benign adnexal tumor demonstrating sebaceous differentiation and affecting the nose, forehead and lateral cheeks. It occurs more commonly in males and presents as a whitish-yellow or skin-colored papule of 2–6 mm, often with central umbilication which differentiates it from basal cell carcinoma (BCC). There is

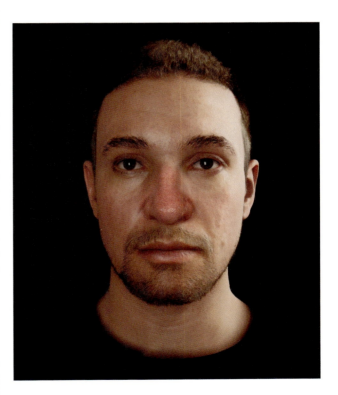

Figure 4.2.9 Patient demonstrating sebaceous hyperplasia in the paranasal area. Note the small yellow, umbilicated lesions. While no treatment is necessary, electrocautery may be effective when requested.

often concomitant seborrhea or telangiectasia. Although benign, it may be cosmetically disturbing or require a biopsy to differentiate it from a BCC [22].

FIBROUS PAPULE

Etiopathogenesis

A fibrous papule (FP) is a benign condition first described in 1965. It commonly occurs as a firm, smooth, dome-shaped, skin-colored papule of 1–5 mm, often presenting singly on the nose [23] (see Figure 4.2.10).

Classically these lesions are hamartomas with unclear pathogenesis, characterized by stellate-shaped stromal cells, multinucleated giant cells and proliferative blood vessels in the dermis. Multiple histologic variants have been described. A biopsy may be necessary to differentiate it from benign adnexal tumors or BCCs [22].

Treatment: Shave or elliptical excision, curettage, electrodesiccation, cryotherapy or laser therapy.

SEBORRHOEIC KERATOSES

Seborrheic keratosis (SK) is one of the most common benign lesions occurring in individuals over 50 years of age. The face is a frequent location, and there is no gender predilection.

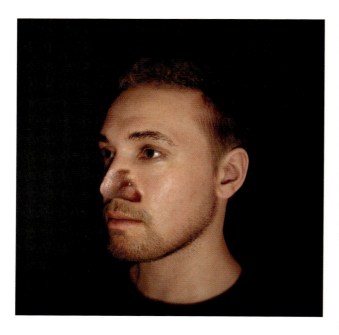

Figure 4.2.10 Middle-aged patient demonstrating a fibrous papule of the nose. Note the smooth, dome-shaped papule demonstrating no overt telangiectasia. FPs commonly occur in middle-aged patients, with no gender predilection. Lesions are typically asymptomatic, with patients often requesting removal for aesthetic reasons.

Etiopathogenesis

Although SKs are considered a sign of aging skin and UV exposure, the exact etiopathogenesis is incompletely understood. Recent oncogenic mutations have been described, but these do not bear a risk of malignant transformation.

SKs are caused by slow maturation of keratinocytes, usually presenting as yellowish circumscribed papules or plaques that may become exophytic, brown or hyperpigmented. Multiple horn pearls are characteristic features. Dermatoscopic features include comedo-like openings, milia-like cysts, fissures and ridges. Histological variants include hyperkeratotic, acanthotic, reticular/adenoid, clonal and irritated subtypes, in addition to melanoacanthoma [24].

Although most SKs are easily identified, they may demonstrate remarkable clinical variability, mimicking lesions such as verrucae, lentigines, actinic keratosis, Bowen's disease, keratoacanthoma and also more aggressive entities such as BCC, squamous cell carcinoma (SCC) and cutaneous melanoma. A small punch biopsy may serve as the differentiating factor [25] (see Figure 4.2.11 a and b).

Treatment: Cryotherapy, curettage and biopsy when warranted by differential diagnosis.

NON-MELANOMA SKIN CANCER

Non-melanoma skin cancer (NMSC) is by far the most frequently diagnosed cancer, with BCC and SCC comprising, respectively, 70% and 25%. BCCs occur most commonly on the face, with the nose being a frequent location (29.7%) [26].

Etiopathogenesis: Actinic keratoses (AKs) are SCC precursors, with a prevalence of more than 40% in the adult population. They share several pathological features with SCC, representing a multistep continuum on chronically sun-exposed fair skin. Normal-appearing skin adjacent to AKs may develop additional AKs due to previous UV exposure and expression of molecular alteration, including p53 mutations, a process termed "field cancerization" [27]. Although no validated parameters are predictive of progression, especially thick AKs should arouse suspicion [28] (see Figures 4.2.12 and 4.2.13).

BASAL CELL CARCINOMA

BCCs occur most commonly on the face, with the nose being a frequent location (29.7%) [26]. Diagnosis of BCC carries an increased risk of developing both new BCC foci and other skin cancer types, including melanoma and SCC. Nodular, superficial and morphoeic subtypes are histologically and clinically differentiated, with new guidelines differentiating "easy-to-treat" and "difficult-to-treat" [29].

SKIN CONDITIONS AFFECTING THE NOSE AND PERINASAL AREA

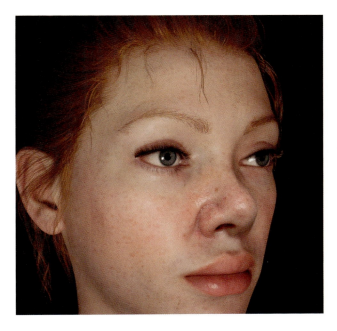

Figure 4.2.11a Patient demonstrating macular seborrheic keratoses of the lateral nose and midface. Note the paranasal telangiectasia secondary to long-standing rosacea.

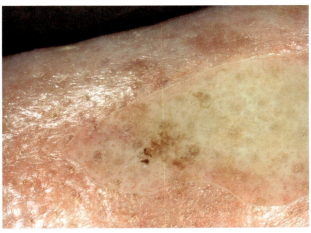

Figure 4.2.11b Dermatoscopic view of a seborrheic keratosis-like lesion showing recent change and irregular peripheral pigmentation. This lesion warrants biopsy to exclude the development of early lentigo maligna.

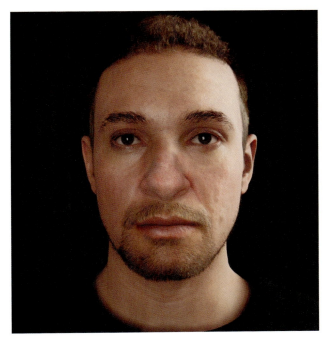

Figure 4.2.12 Actinic and seborrheic keratoses in a patient with widespread actinic damage and previous squamous cell carcinomas of the face.

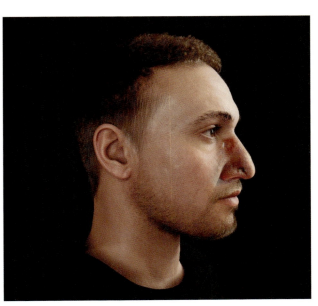

Figure 4.2.13 Patient demonstrating a squamous cell carcinoma on the lateral nose. Importantly, these lesions may metastasize, and careful multidisciplinary management is advised. Note the adjacent curettage scar from a previous BCC.

Although there may be various pathogenetic factors in the development of both NMSC and melanoma, chronic exposure to UV radiation (sunlight and tanning beds) is considered the most important [15] (see Figures 4.2.14–4.2.16).

MALIGNANT MELANOMA (MM)

Etiopathogenesis

Melanoma constitutes a highly virulent malignant tumor arising from melanocytes. Although comprising approximately 4% of skin cancer cases, it is a deadly disease accounting for 75% of skin cancer deaths [30]. Early stages may be successfully treated by adequate surgery of lesional and perilesional skin, but metastases portend a

Table 4.2.3 Presentation of Non-Melanoma Skin Cancer

	AK	SCC	BCC
Incidence	40% adult population 0.025–16%/year evolve to SCC	20% of NMSC	75% of NMSC
↑ Prevalence (20 years)	No data	133%	35%
Development	Continuum with SCC "field cancerization"	Continuum with actinic keratoses	Arise de novo
		++ recurrence	↑ Risk new foci/other SCC/MM
Metastases	No data	0.1–4%	Rare
			Least aggressive NMSC

AK: actinic keratosis; BCC: basal cell carcinoma; MM: malignant melanoma; NMSC: non-melanoma skin cancer; SCC: squamous cell carcinoma.

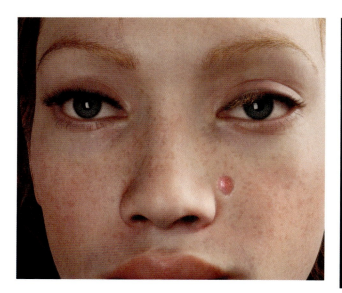

Figure 4.2.14 Patient with BCC of the lateral nose. Note the classical appearance of a pearly papule with telangiectasia.

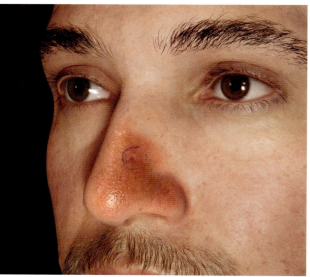

Figure 4.2.15 Patient demonstrating a nodular BCC referred for Moh's surgery after small biopsy demonstrating an infiltrative growth pattern. Note the characteristic pearly border and telangiectasia.

significant drop in survival rates, making early and correct diagnosis imperative. Early misdiagnosis, which significantly reduces survival, accounts for more pathology and dermatology malpractice claims than any other skin condition. Clinical vigilance and early biopsy are critical.

The classically described histological variants include lentigo maligna melanoma, superficial spreading melanoma and nodular melanoma. Acral lentiginous, mucosal, desmoplastic and nevoid melanoma have also been described [31,32].

Although less common than NMSC, melanoma may occur on the nasal skin, septum and mucosa. The classical appearance is that of a pigmented lesion demonstrating three or more of the following:

A: **A**symmetry
B: **B**order irregularity
C: **C**olors >3
D: **D**iameter >6 mm

Any new pigmented lesion should be critically appraised, as the majority of melanomas arise de novo and not in an existing melanocytic nevus. However, constant change in an existing lesion also warrants biopsy.

Extreme clinical vigilance and multidisciplinary management are critical given the potentially grave prognosis and frequently extensive surgery [30] (see Figure 4.2.17).

Management: Surgery is usually the treatment of choice, with excision according to Breslow depth. In follow-up, regular total cutaneous examination, with frequency dictated by the histological depth of the primary lesion, is mandatory. Multidisciplinary collaboration is advised in the management of this patient cohort.

SKIN CONDITIONS AFFECTING THE NOSE AND PERINASAL AREA

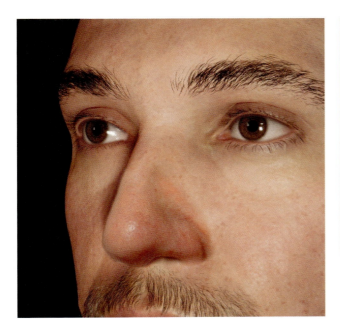

Figure 4.2.16a Patient demonstrating an annular morphoeic BCC in the right paranasal region. This new patient presented late due to the fact that she equated the lesion to a residue from a previous filler procedure.

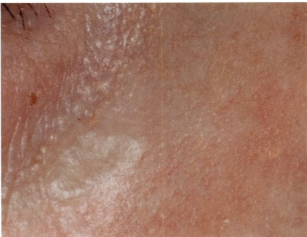

Figure 4.2.16b Close-up view of Figure 4.2.16a. Note the raised, pearly lesional border. Although these lesions may be insidious, they mandate early detection. Due to infiltration depth, this patient required extensive surgery.

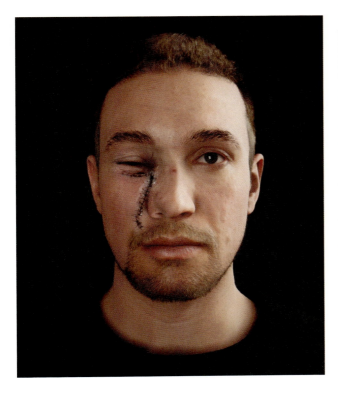

Figure 4.2.16c Postsurgical appearance directly after Moh's surgery. Note the extent of the scar.

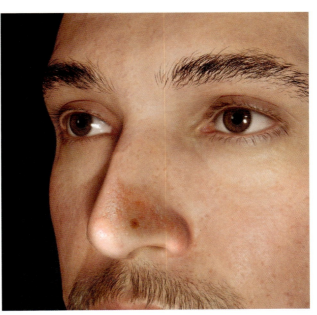

Figure 4.2.17 Lentigo maligna melanoma of the lateral nose. The presentation of these lesions may be slow and insidious. A biopsy is critical for any new or evolving pigmented lesion.

CONCLUSION

Although cutaneous manifestations of the nose and perinasal region in patients presenting for non-surgical rhinoplasty may be subtle, the timeous and optimal treatment of these conditions is imperative in order to prevent further complicating an intrinsically high-risk procedure.

Multispecialty collaboration is often helpful in optimizing early diagnosis of subtle variants and current treatment nuances.

BIBLIOGRAPHY

1. Heydenrych I, Kapoor KM, Boulle K De, Goodman G, Swift A, Kumar N. A 10-point plan for avoiding hyaluronic acid dermal filler-related complications during facial aesthetic procedures and algorithms for management. Clin Cosmet Investig Dermatol. 2018;(11):603–611.
2. Kosins AM, Obagi ZE. Managing the difficult soft tissue envelope in facial and rhinoplasty surgery. Aesthetic Surg J. 2017;37(2):143–157.
3. Heydenrych I, De Boulle K, Kapoor KM, Bertossi D. The 10-point plan 2021: updated concepts for improved procedural safety during facial filler treatments. Clin Cosmet Investig Dermatol. 2021;14:779.
4. Whitley R, Baines J. Clinical management of herpes simplex virus infections: past, present, and future. F1000Research. 2018;7(1).
5. Sakr A, Brégeon F, Mège J-L, Rolain J-M, Blin O. Staphylococcus aureus nasal colonization: an update on mechanisms, epidemiology, risk factors, and subsequent infections. Front Microbiol. 2018;9:2419.
6. D'Cunha NM, Peterson GM, Baby KE, Thomas J. Impetigo: a need for new therapies in a world of increasing antimicrobial resistance. J Clin Pharm Ther. 2017;43(1):150–153.
7. Sassmannshausen R, Deurenberg RH, Köck R, Hendrix R, Jurke A, Rossen JWA, et al. MRSA prevalence and associated risk factors among health-care workers in non-outbreak situations in the Dutch-German EUREGIO. Front Microbiol. 2016;7:1273.
8. McLaughlin J, Watterson S, Layton AM, Bjourson AJ, Barnard E, McDowell A. Propionibacterium acnes and acne vulgaris: new insights from the integration of population genetic, multi-omic, biochemical and host-microbe studies. Microorganisms. 2019;7(5):128.
9. Zaenglein AL, Pathy AL, Schlosser BJ, Alikhan A, Baldwin HE, Berson DS, et al. Guidelines of care for the management of acne vulgaris. J Am Acad Dermatol. 2016;74(5):945–973.
10. Feldman SR, Tan J, Poulin Y, Dirschka T, Kerrouche N, Manna V. The efficacy of adapalene-benzoyl peroxide combination increases with number of acne lesions. J Am Acad Dermatol. 2011;64(6):1085–1091.
11. Thiboutot D, Anderson R, Cook-Bolden F, Draelos Z, Gallo RL, Granstein RD, et al. Standard management options for rosacea: the 2019 update by the National Rosacea Society Expert Committee. J Am Acad Dermatol. 2020;82(6):1501–1510.
12. Cobo R, Vitery L. Isotretinoin use in thick-skinned rhinoplasty patients. Facial Plast Surg. 2016;32(06):656–661.
13. Medgyesi B, Dajnoki Z, Béke G, Gáspár K, Szabó IL, Janka EA, et al. Rosacea is characterized by a profoundly diminished skin barrier. J Invest Dermatol. 2020;140(10):1938–1950.
14. Baldwin H, Alexis AF, Andriessen A, Berson DS, Farris P, Harper J, et al. Evidence of barrier deficiency in rosacea and the importance of integrating OTC skincare products into treatment regimens. J Drugs Dermatology JDD. 2021;20(4):384–392.
15. Searle T, Ali FR, Al-Niaimi F. Perioral dermatitis: diagnosis, proposed etiologies, and management. J Cosmet Dermatol. 2021;20(12):3839–3848.
16. Chopra K, Calva D, Sosin M, Tadisina KK, Banda A, De La Cruz C, et al. A comprehensive examination of topographic thickness of skin in the human face. Aesthetic Surg J. 2015;35(8):1007–1013.
17. Warshaw EM, Schlarbaum JP, Maibach HI, Silverberg JI, Taylor JS, Atwater AR, et al. Facial dermatitis in male patients referred for patch testing: retrospective analysis of north American contact dermatitis group data, 1994 to 2016. JAMA Dermatology. 2020;156(1):79–84.
18. Del Rosso JQ, Kircik LH. The integration of physiologically-targeted skin care in the management of atopic dermatitis: focus on the use of a cleanser and moisturizer system incorporating a ceramide precursor, filaggrin degradation products, and specific "skin-barrier-friendly" ex. J Drugs Dermatology JDD. 2013;12(7):s85–91.
19. Sanders MGH, Pardo LM, Franco OH, Ginger RS, Nijsten T. Prevalence and determinants of seborrhoeic dermatitis in a middle-aged and elderly population: the rotterdam study. Br J Dermatol. 2018;178(1):148–153.
20. Kamamoto CSL, Nishikaku AS, Gompertz OF, Melo AS, Hassun KM, Bagatin E. Cutaneous fungal microbiome: malassezia yeasts in seborrheic dermatitis scalp in a randomized, comparative and therapeutic trial. Dermatoendocrinol. 2017;9(1):e1361573.
21. Abbas Z, Ghodsi SZ, Abedeni R. Effect of itraconazole on the quality of life in patients with moderate to severe seborrheic dermatitis: a randomized, placebo-controlled trial. Dermatol Pract Concept. 2016;6(3):11.
22. Sand M, Sand D, Thrandorf C, Paech V, Altmeyer P, Bechara FG. Cutaneous lesions of the nose. Head Face Med. 2010;6(1):1–16.
23. Chan J-YL, Wang K-H, Fang C-L, Chen W-Y. Fibrous papule of the face, similar to tuberous sclerosis complex-associated angiofibroma, shows activation of the mammalian target of rapamycin pathway: evidence for a novel therapeutic strategy? PLoS One. 2014;9(2):e89467.
24. Wollina U. Seborrheic keratoses: the most common benign skin tumor of humans: clinical presentation and an update on pathogenesis and treatment options. Open Access Maced J Med Sci. 2018;6(11):2270.
25. Li W-R, Lin L. Seborrheic keratosis in a young woman: a mimicker of keratoacanthoma. Int J Dermatology Venereol. 2020;3(02):116–117.
26. Ciążyńska M, Kamińska-Winciorek G, Lange D, Lewandowski B, Reich A, Sławińska M, et al. The incidence and clinical analysis of non-melanoma skin cancer. Sci Rep. 2021;11(1):1–10.
27. Didona D, Paolino G, Bottoni U, Cantisani C. Non melanoma skin cancer pathogenesis overview. Biomedicines. 2018;6(1):6.

28. Heerfordt IM, Poulsen T, Wulf HC. Actinic keratoses contiguous with squamous cell carcinomas are mostly non-hyperkeratotic and with severe dysplasia. J Clin Pathol. 2021.
29. Peris K, Fargnoli MC, Garbe C, Kaufmann R, Bastholt L, Seguin NB, et al. Diagnosis and treatment of basal cell carcinoma: European consensus-based interdisciplinary guidelines. Eur J Cancer. 2019;118:10–34.
30. Davis LE, Shalin SC, Tackett AJ. Current state of melanoma diagnosis and treatment. Cancer Biol Ther. 2019;20(11):1366–1379.
31. Iznardo H, Garcia-Melendo C, Yélamos O. Lentigo maligna: clinical presentation and appropriate management. Clin Cosmet Investig Dermatol. 2020;13:837.
32. Samaniego E, Redondo P. Lentigo maligno. Actas Dermo-Sifiliográficas. 2013;104(9):757–775.

CHAPTER **4.3**

Conditions Affecting the Nose and Perinasal Skin and Their Assessment and Diagnosis

Ilaria Proietti

In a day-to-day practice, the pretreatment assessment is crucial to avoid possible adverse effects of the filler treatment. Patients can present with various cutaneous conditions affecting the nose and perinasal skin. Some of the conditions, e.g., active rosacea, can deteriorate the skin barrier function even a few weeks after apparent clearing, significantly increasing the risk of complications [1]. Infections in or adjacent to the treated region can lead to contamination by infectious organisms at the filler site. Consequently, patients may develop multiple red, tender nodules as well as signs and symptoms of infection. In case of a single facial abscess, it is probable that contamination occurred during the injection, whereas if a patient presents with multiple abscesses, it is likely that the contents of the syringe were inquinated. Less frequently, diffuse granulomatous inflammation may appear as a result of systemic response [2]. Thus, in patients with an ongoing skin disorder, the rhinofiller procedure should be postponed and a proper treatment should be planned [3].

Nowadays, we have many tools at our disposal to assess and diagnose skin conditions before eventual filler procedure.

Dermoscopy (known as epiluminescence microscopy and skin surface microscopy) is a non-invasive, in vivo technique performed with a handled instrument called a dermatoscope. The examination allows one to visualize the skin structures in the epidermis, at the dermoepidermal junction, and in the upper dermis, normally invisible to the naked eye [4, 5]. The analysis of dermoscopic patterns permits one to establish a diagnosis of melanocytic and inflammatory lesions [6].

Optical coherence tomography (OCT) is an advanced, non-invasive, optical imaging technique that uses low-power infrared light to picture up to 2 mm below the skin surface. The practitioner can obtain real-time, precise, high-resolution information about the skin microstructure and the exact depth of skin layers and structures [7]. OCT is a useful instrument in diagnosing skin cancers, helping to avoid unnecessary skin biopsies; it has been shown to facilitate the assessment of inflammatory diseases such as acne, atopic dermatitis, seborrheic dermatitis, and aesthetic skin evaluation [7–17].

Recently, a **speckle-variance OCT** (dynamic OCT; D-OCT) was developed. It relies on detecting motion in the OCT images and enables the visualization of vascular architecture and the blood flow of the skin [8].

Line-field confocal optical coherence tomography (LC-OCT), another new variant of OCT, allows vertical and horizontal skin imaging with high resolution close to conventional histopathology [9, 10]. Although only a few studies on its use in cutaneous disorders have been reported up to now [10–12], in some cases it demonstrated an excellent correlation with conventional histopathology [11].

Reflectance confocal microscopy (RCM) is a non-invasive, in vivo imaging method that enables visualization of the epidermis and superficial dermis in real time. This technique involves the formation of reflected light under laser excitation, which performs tomographic scanning on cells or tissues. The signal is subsequently imaged by the computer with a resolution that might be comparable to conventional histology. RCM has been shown to be useful in the diagnosis of pigmentary diseases, inflammatory diseases, skin tumors, and other common skin diseases [18, 19].

Rosacea is a common chronic disease that can be characterized by a variety of cutaneous and ocular manifestations. Cutaneous signs primarily involve the central face, with findings such as persistent centrofacial redness, papules, pustules, flushing, telangiectasia, and phymatous skin changes (e.g., rhinophyma). Ocular manifestations include lid margin telangiectasias, conjunctival injection, ocular irritation, and other signs and symptoms.

CONDITIONS AFFECTING THE NOSE AND PERINASAL SKIN

The pathogenesis of rosacea is complex and still poorly understood. Among the suggested contributing factors which have been described, there are abnormalities in immunity, inflammatory reactions to cutaneous microorganisms, vascular dysfunction, ultraviolet light exposure, and genetic factors.

Demodex folliculorum is a saprophytic mite that inhabits sebaceous follicles and can be found in the normal skin in almost all adults. Nevertheless, increased density of *Demodex* mites in patients with rosacea has been reported in multiple studies [20–22]. A massive *Demodex* infestation makes the patient incompatible for treatment, as the parasite can populate the site of injection. Furthermore, an augmented inflammatory state of active rosacea is a contraindication to the filler [3]. In the treatment of rosacea, it is important to allow a sufficient skin barrier restoration before filler injection. Such a process may require 3–4 weeks after apparent clearance [23].

In **dermoscopy**, an erythematotelangiectatic type of rosacea is represented by the presence of linear, violaceous vessels characteristically arranged in a polygonal network (vascular polygons) [24] (see Figure 4.3.1). Additional characteristics include rosettes [25], follicular plugs, white/yellowish scales, orange-yellowish areas (granulomatous rosacea), dilated follicles, and follicular pustules (papulopustular rosacea) [26].

Rosacea is often accompanied by a high density of *D. folliculorum* (demodicosis). Typical dermoscopic feature of demodicosis are demodex tails—gelatinous, whitish, creamy threads and follicular gray dots [27, 28].

In **D-OCT,** erythema is visualized as small, dotted vessels in superficial skin layers and, in the deeper parts, the telangiectasia presents with a network of vessels with a larger diameter than in normal skin. D-OCT also enables the assessment of treatment with vasoconstricting topical agents and laser. After dye laser therapy, a former broad vascular network is replaced by a fuzzy appearance of the vessels [8].

The **RCM** technique enables the diagnosis and monitoring of treatment of rosacea. The items of interest are *Demodex* mites which manifest as roundish/elongated, cone-shaped, gray structures surrounded by a bright ring. Patients affected by rosacea, especially the papulopustular type, show significantly higher mite numbers than healthy subjects [29, 30]. The reduction of the *Demodex* population after topical treatment may be correlated with clinical improvement [31, 32].

Active herpes infection: The global prevalence of herpes simplex virus type 1 (HSV-1) infection in the population under the age of 50 reaches approximately 67% [33]. HSV-1 is transmitted during close contact from person to person through secretions containing the virus. After primary infection, HSV-1 institutes chronic infection in

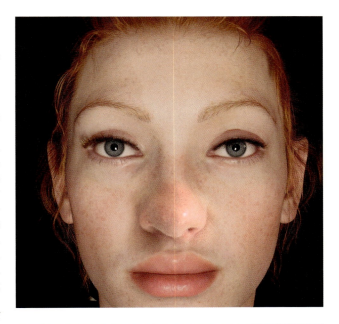

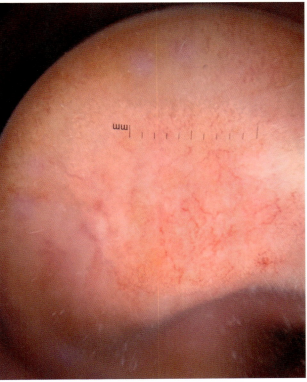

Figure 4.3.1 Clinical (a) and dermatoscopic (b, 30×) characteristics of telangiectatic rosacea.

sensory ganglia and reactivates on mucosa and skin. Even if the recurrent infections are frequently asymptomatic, they can produce a variety of signs and symptoms. These include lesions that involve the mucosa and/or skin, e.g., oral and perioral lesions ("cold sores"), which can extend to the nasal and perinasal region; genital lesions; and ocular infections (e.g., herpetic keratitis). In rare cases this can lead to serious systemic disorders such as encephalitis and neonatal multiorgan disease.

In case of evident active HSV infection, filler treatment should be postponed and an antiviral therapy prescribed (acyclovir, valaciclovir, or famciclovir). These drugs can prevent contamination at the injection site, the reactivation of infection, and the spread of HSV [3].

The injection trauma and dermal fillers are thought to be a possible trigger of herpetic lesions [34]. Thus, in patients with a known history of frequent HSV reactivations, a prophylactic antiviral treatment should be considered [3].

Dermoscopy: Although the diagnosis of the infection is usually based on the anamnesis and clinic evaluation, its dermatoscopic features have been described and can be particularly helpful in questionable cases. These include central brown pigmentation surrounded by a whitish hue and peripheral erythema [35] (see Figure 4.3.2).

RCM enables detection of cytopathic effects of herpes simplex in the skin. The RCM image shows the intraepidermal cavities with acantholytic cells admixed with pleomorphic large keratinocytes along with multinucleated giant cells corresponding to keratinocytes infected by HSV [36].

Although **LC-OCT** is a very advanced but not yet universally accessible technique, it may represent a further advancement in the non-invasive diagnosis of different cutaneous disorders such as herpes infection. The available studies show some common features of HSV presence in the skin: well-defined, intraepidermal, roundish, dark areas corresponding to the vesicular spaces. The largest, roundish elements likely corresponded to giant, ballooning, and multinucleated cells floating inside the vesicles along with acantholytic keratinocytes and inflammatory cells [37].

Compared with RCM, LC-OCT enables the vertical view, showing the precise blister size and localization in the epidermis, with clear visualization of depth and contours [37].

Acne is a common, chronic, or recurrent disorder characterized by the presence of papules, pustules, or nodules on the face, neck, and trunk. The pathogenesis of acne vulgaris consists of the interaction of multiple factors such as follicular hyperkeratinization, increased sebum production, and C*utibacterium acnes* (formerly *Propionibacterium acnes*, an anaerobic bacterium that is a normal component of skin flora) [38]. All of these lead to the development of inflammation and formation of comedones. Typically, acne affects adolescents and young adults but is not limited to these ages. Skin involvement can present with various grades of severity, from minimal involvement to disfiguring and highly inflammatory lesions.

In patients with active acne *C. acnes* induces a cytokine-mediated inflammation. Additionally, the elevated number of resistant *C. acnes* on the borders of topically treated acne areas predispose to the development of biofilms, which are known for playing a role in filler complications. It is important to be aware of the "safe distance" between the acne area and filler injection site, which cannot be determined [2, 23, 39].

The biofilm acts as a "fortress", which protects the bacteria from antibacterial agents. All kinds of implants, including fillers, favor the contamination and subsequent infection. Once the biofilm develops, neither the immune system nor medications can invade the barrier. It is very difficult, or even impossible, to destroy the bacterial colonies until the filler is removed. Biofilm binds irreversibly to injected material [2, 39].

In consideration of conditions, a proper treatment should be introduced before the decision to use filler. In order to let the skin barrier restore, future injections should be postponed by 3–4 weeks after apparent clearance [23] (see Figure 4.3.3).

OCT has been used to examine acne morphology [40] and monitor acne skin in real time [40, 41]. The investigation of infundibular regions of pilosebaceous units and acne lesion subtypes identified enlarged sebaceous glands and enabled the acne subtype distinction (closed and open comedones, papules, and pustules) [40]. The OCT image may show the acne lesion borders and differentiate alterations of the skin induced by collagen or other tissue damage induced by inflammation. D-OCT showed that the vessels in the acne region are coarse and less organized than those in the surrounding normal tissue [41].

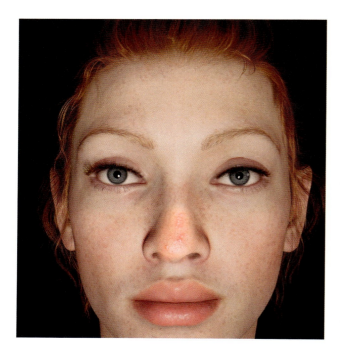

Figure 4.3.2 Second-day nasal herpes simplex (blisters).

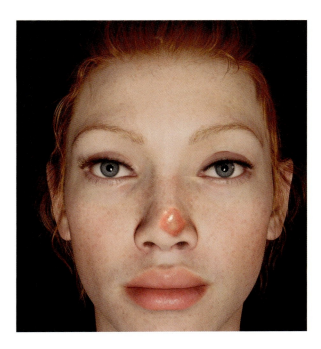

Figure 4.3.3 Acne lesions (comedones, papules and nodules).

RCM gives the possibility of in vivo identification of principal histopathologic characteristics of different acne lesions and the subclinical alterations present in apparently healthy skin of acne patients [42]. The RCM images collected during the studies showed that hair follicles of acne patients were enlarged with hyperkeratinized borders and sebum plugs compared to hair follicles in healthy skin. The concomitant inflammatory component was also described in relation to papules and pustules [42, 43]. Additionally the studies support the hypothesis that follicles of acne skin are different from healthy follicles, as the quantity of enlarged, hyperkeratinized follicles decreased after topical acne treatment [42].

Impetigo is a superficial bacterial skin infection caused by *Streptococcus pyogenes* and *Staphylococcus aureus*, typically observed in children; however, adults can also be affected. It may be divided into primary impetigo (bacterial invasion of previously normal skin) and secondary impetigo (infection in areas of underlying skin disorders such as abrasions, insect bites, or conditions such as eczema). The occurrence of secondary impetigo is sometimes described as "impetiginization". It is clinically characterized by fragile vesicles, pustules, or bullae on an erythematous base which easily rupture and cover over with honey-colored crusts. Most commonly, lesions appear on the face (especially the nose and mouth) and extremities [44].

The pyogenic bacteria have a high contaminating potential. These not only can create resistant biofilms [2, 45, 46] but naturally produce hyaluronidases, which allow a rapid and widespread invasion of the tissues [2]. Thus, in patients with an active infection, filler injections should be postponed and a proper treatment should be introduced. In those with underlying *S. aureus* carrier status, therapy with an intranasal topical antibiotic (mupirocin, neomycin, bacitracin) or antibacterial agent (chlorhexidine or bleach baths) could be considered [47].

Additionally, correct preinjection skin preparation appears to be crucial to avoid the infection, as *S. aureus* biofilm can cause contamination despite standard antimicrobial procedures [48].

Dermoscopy: Dermatoscopic images present with peripheral scaling, yellow crusts, and dotted vessels [28].

RCM: Although the diagnosis of impetigo is usually clinical, confocal microscopy could be helpful for its early diagnosis. The microscopic picture may demonstrate superficial subcorneal acantholysis and the presence of small bright inflammatory cells [49] (see Figure 4.3.4).

Seborrheic dermatitis is a chronic, relapsing dermatitis that affects infants and adults. The gravity may vary from minimal, asymptomatic desquamation of the scalp (dandruff) to more extensive involvement. Seborrheic dermatitis has been associated with HIV infection, Parkinson disease, neurologic disorders, and use of neuroleptic medications. The pathogenesis of seborrheic dermatitis is not completely understood. It is correlated with proliferation of *Malassezia* yeast (a saprophyte of normal skin), which metabolizes skin lipids. Both the fungus and its metabolites have a proinflammatory potential stimulating a host immune response [50]. Clinically, seborrheic dermatitis is characterized by well-demarcated, erythematous plaques with greasy-looking, yellowish scales diffused in regions rich in sebaceous glands: the scalp, external ear, center of face, upper part of the trunk, and intertriginous areas (see Figure 4.3.5).

Filler treatment should be postponed in the case of active seborrheic dermatitis due to the risk of a high density of *Malassezia*, which has a positive correlation with the severity of dermatitis manifestations [1, 51]. Such conditions could result in contamination of the injection site and further posttreatment complications. Additionally, an important inflammation of the skin, for its part, can be considered as a contraindication to filler treatment [1].

Dermoscopy: The classical dermoscopic findings include dotted vessels in a patchy distribution and fine yellowish scales, sometimes in combination with white scales. Follicular plugs, orange-yellowish areas, whitish structureless areas, and linear branching vessels are less common features [5, 6] (see Figure 4.3.5).

OCT: Although seborrheic dermatitis is diagnosed primarily through a naked eye examination by the clinician or with use of the dermatoscope, the OCT investigation may be helpful in difficult cases. The OCT image shows a higher density of sebaceous glands, and the papillary dermis appears relatively darker in comparison with healthy skin [52]. The D-OCT scan of seborrheic

NON-SURGICAL RHINOPLASTY

dermatitis of the scalp shows a transition in vasculature from the superficial to the deep plexus. The superficial plexus reveals small, dilated vessels exchanging with thinner arborizing vessels, while the deep plexus demonstrates "lavalike" dilated arborizing vessels organized in a netlike distribution. The elongation of perpendicular vessel columns and dilations of the deep plexus may be observed [53].

RCM: Similarly to the OCT, the confocal microscopy may be used in difficult, questionable cases. Typical features of seborrheic dermatitis are thickening of the stratum corneum and coexisting highly refractive, round to polygonal structures corresponding to parakeratosis, spongiosis, and peculiar horizontal orientation of dilated blood vessels in the upper dermis, usually located around adnexal structures. Due to concomitant seborrhea, *D. folliculorum* may be detected inside sebaceous glands [54, 55].

Lichen planus is a rare chronic inflammatory condition involving the skin and/or mucosa. It most commonly affects middle-aged adults. The typical clinical presentation of cutaneous lichen planus consists of papulosquamous eruption of flat-topped, violaceous, and pruriginous papules.

Psoriasis is a common chronic inflammatory skin disease that may present with a variety of clinical manifestations. Globally, it affects around 2–4% of males and females. Psoriasis is observed in adolescents and adults; however, children can also be affected. The most common subtype of psoriasis is characterized by chronic, well-demarcated, erythematous plaques with overlying, coarse scale.

Both entities are characterized by the Koebner phenomenon, an isomorphic response which describes the appearance of new skin lesions of a preexisting dermatosis on areas of cutaneous injury. In patients with active lichen planus or psoriasis, trauma caused by injection can provoke an exacerbation and spread of lesions [56]. Thus, proper therapy should be introduced before filler treatment to avoid such complications (see Figure 4.3.6).

DERMOSCOPY

Lichen planus: The dermoscopic hallmarks are the Wickham striae, which usually present as pearly whitish reticular structures. Additional dermoscopic characteristics include dotted, globular, and/or linear vessels, mainly localized at the periphery of the lesion; violet, reddish, pink, brown, or yellow background; white/yellow dots; and some pigmented structures [5].

Psoriasis: Classical features consist of diffuse white scales and symmetrical and regular dotted vessels on a red background. The presence of important hyperkeratosis may impede the view of underlying features. In such cases, scale removal may reveal the vascular pattern as well as possible tiny red blood drops (known as the dermoscopic "Auspitz sign") [5].

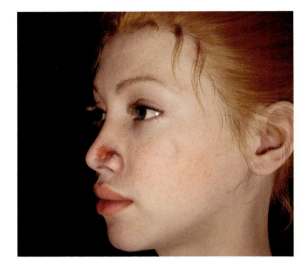
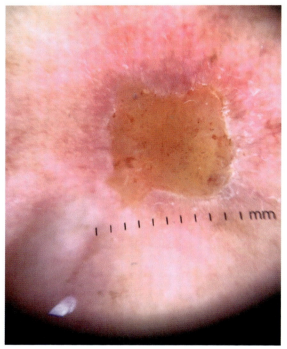

Figure 4.3.4 Clinical (a) and dermatoscopic (b, 30×) features of impetigo arising after cryotherapy for actinic keratosis of the nose.

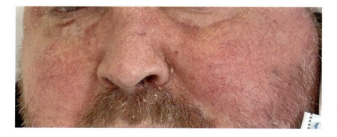

Figure 4.3.5 Clinical features of seborrheic dermatitis in HIV-infected patient.

CONDITIONS AFFECTING THE NOSE AND PERINASAL SKIN

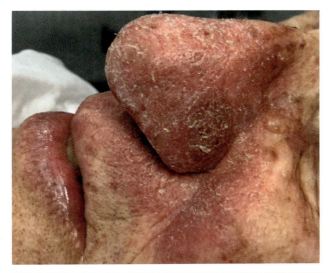

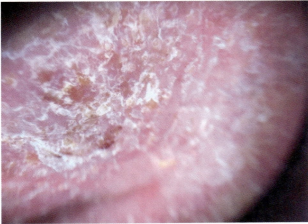

Figure 4.3.6 Clinical (a) and dermatoscopic (b, 30×) features of severe psoriasis of the face.

Psoriasis: The OCT examination enables one to visualize typical features of psoriatic skin, which include hyperkeratosis, acanthosis, pronounced regular rete ridges, and dilated vessels in the dermis with components of inflammation, proliferation of the epidermis, and angiogenesis, which contribute to the development of psoriasis. In addition, the D-OCT technique allows one to picture the typical vessel capillary loops (spikes) in the papillary dermis. The measurement of epidermal thickness appears to be useful in estimating the severity of psoriasis [8, 59].

REFLECTANCE CONFOCAL MICROSCOPY

Lichen planus: The confocal microscopy examination reveals features typical for interface dermatitis, such as epidermal disarray, hypergranulosis, spongiosis, and necrotic keratinocytes. The dermis, in its superficial layer, presents with diffuse inflammatory infiltrate of highly refractive lymphocytes, which tends to blur or even mask the annular structure of dermal papillae. Melanophages and dilatated blood vessels may be also found [60, 61].

Psoriasis: In clinical practice, in questionable cases histological examination is required to define the diagnosis, set up a proper therapy, and determine timing of the follow-up examinations. The RCM imaging allows elucidating the major key microscopic features of psoriasis in real time, without surgical intervention, and with a very good correlation with conventional histology. Typical features which can be found in psoriatic skin are parakeratosis, reduction or absence of the granular layer, papillomatosis, acanthosis with normal honeycomb pattern of epidermis, and dilated vessels in the upper dermis [62]. A careful examination may be helpful in distinguishing psoriasis from other inflammatory diseases such as seborrheic dermatitis [55]. RCM resulted in effective monitoring of treatment response in psoriasis [63–65].

OPTICAL COHERENCE TOMOGRAPHY

Lichen planus: Although the OCT technique is still very innovative, the possibility of visualization of some of the important lichen characteristics has been described. Those include irregular acanthosis with increased epidermal layer thickness, sawtooth appearance of the dermo-epidermal interline, focal hypergranulosis, and the typical interface inflammatory infiltrate, seen as effacement of the DEJ interline. Other manifestations possible to see in high-resolution images are basal vacuolar degeneration represented by total obliteration of the ringlike structures around the dermal papillae and inflammatory and necrotic cells in the epidermis seen as bright spots. These aspects allow the differentiation in vivo between lichen planus and other inflammatory diseases (psoriasis, eczema) [57, 58].

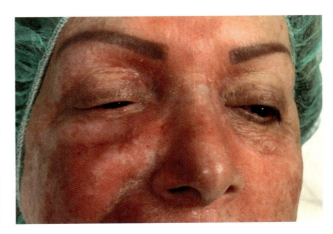

Figure 4.3.7 Patient with lupus.

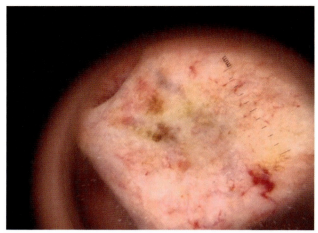
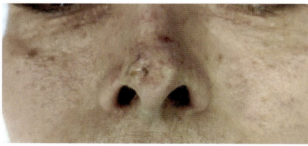

Figure 4.3.8 Clinical (a) and dermatoscopic (b, 30×) features of scleroderma of the nose (atrophy, telangiectasias and petechiae).

Autoimmune diseases (e.g., active morphea, systemic lupus, scleroderma, rheumatoid arthritis): Some practitioners prefer to avoid injectable treatments in patients with active autoimmune disorders because of their concern of disease reactivation via antigenic stimulation. Despite this theoretical risk, there is no causal relationship between the use of fillers and disease reactivation phenomenon [66, 67]. Additionally, the literature reports cases of hyaluronic acid treatment in patients affected by lupus with satisfactory results and no adverse reactions or disease aggravation [68] (see Figures 4.3.7 and 4.3.8).

Thus, the decision of filler treatment in patients with autoimmune diseases should be evaluated on a case-by-case basis.

COMPUTED TOMOGRAPHY

Computed tomography (CT) is an advanced, non-invasive imaging technique used to acquire detailed internal images of the body. CT scanners use a rotating x-ray tube and a row of detectors to estimate x-ray attenuations by different tissues.

The CT scan is frequently used to diagnose nose disorders and evaluate the anatomical structure before performing medical procedures (e.g., septoplasty, reconstructions of nasal malformations) [69–71]. Although in patients treated with filler, its use is still not very common, along with magnetic resonance imaging (MRI) and positron emission tomography (PET)-CT, it could be considered a valid option for pretreatment evaluation and/or diagnosis of filler complications.

CT may be helpful to assess the dorsal status of the nose, which can be classified in straight, hump, and pseudohump, as well as concomitant septal deviation and other nose malformations affecting the general aspect and functionality [72].

In the evaluation of filler treatment, MRI is superior to a CT, as it allows assessment of soft tissues. The most important advantage of CT is the identification of calcifications, which can be found in some of the fillers and filler-related complications. Additionally, contrast-enhanced CT is preferred in the suspicion of infectious complications [73].

Cholesteryl hyaluronic acid (CHA) is made of microparticles of bonelike substance suspended in an aqueous sodium carboxymethyl cellulose gel. This can be used to treat, for example, marionette lines or nasolabial folds. The CHA filler tends to evoke a foreign body reaction and nodule formation. The CT scan reveals the CHA as well-defined linear streaks or rounded masses (clumps of calcification). All other types of fillers do not show any calcifications unless they provoke a foreign body reaction—a foreign body granuloma can be identified by eggshell calcifications. Some fillers (especially permanent ones, e.g., silicone) can provoke a severe chronic inflammatory thickening of the soft tissues resulting in scarring and disfigurement. In these cases, the CT scan may show a thick bandlike subcutaneous deposition.

BIBLIOGRAPHY

1. Heydenrych I, De Boulle K, Kapoor KM, Bertossi D. The 10-point plan 2021: updated concepts for improved procedural safety during facial filler treatments. Clin Cosmet Investig Dermatol. 2021 Jul 6;14:779–814.
2. DeLorenzi C. Complications of injectable fillers, part I. Aesthet Surg J. 2013.
3. De Boulle K, Heydenrych I, Patient factors influencing dermal filler complications: prevention, assessment, and treatment. Clin Cosmet Investig Dermatol. 2015 Apr 15;8:205–14.
4. Kaushik A, Natsis N, Gordon SC, Seiverling EV. A practical review of dermoscopy for pediatric dermatology part I: melanocytic growths. Pediatr Dermatol. 2020 Sep;37(5): 789–797. doi: 10.1111/pde.14291. Epub 2020 Aug 4.
5. Sgouros D, Apalla Z, Ioannides D, Katoulis A, Rigopoulos D, Sotiriou E, Stratigos A, Vakirlis E, Lallas A. Dermoscopy of common inflammatory disorders. Dermatol Clin. 2018 Oct;36(4):359–368. doi: 10.1016/j.det.2018.05.003. Epub 2018 Jul.

6. Lallas A, Argenziano G, Apalla Z, et al. Dermoscopic patterns of common facial inflammatory skin diseases. J Eur Acad Dermatol Venereol. 2014;28:609–614.
7. Kislevitz M, Akgul Y, Wamsley C et al. Use of Optical Coherence Tomography (OCT) in Aesthetic Skin Assessment – A Short Review. Lasers Surg Med. 2020 Oct;52(8):699–704.
8. Schuh S, Holmes J, Ulrich M et al. Imaging Blood Vessel Morphology in Skin: Dynamic Optical Coherence Tomography as a Novel Potential Diagnostic Tool in Dermatology. Dermatol Ther (Heidelb). 2017 Jun;7(2):187–202.
9. Dubois A, Levecq O, Azimani H, et al. Line-field confocal optical coherence tomography for high-resolution noninvasive imaging of skin tumors. J Biomed Opt. 2018;23:1–9.
10. Ruini C, Schuh S, Pellacani G, French L, Welzel J, Sattler E. In vivo imaging of sarcoptes scabiei infestation using line-field confocal optical coherence tomography. J Eur Acad Dermatol Venereol. 2020;34:e808–e809.
11. Ruini C, Schuh S, Sattler E, Welzel J. Line-field confocal optical coherence tomography-practical applications in dermatology and comparison with established imaging methods. Skin Res Technol. 2020. https://doi.org/10.1111/srt.12949. Epub ahead of print.
12. Tognetti L, Fiorani D, Cinotti E, Rubegni P. Tridimensional skin imaging in aquagenic keratoderma: virtual histology by line-field confocal optical coherence tomography. Int J Dermatol. 2021;60:e52–e54.
13. Forsea AM, Carstea EM, Ghervase L, Giurcaneanu C, Pavelescu G. Clinical application of optical coherence tomography for the imaging of non-melanocytic cutaneous tumors: a pilot multi-modal study. J Med Life. 2010 Oct–Dec;3(4):381–389. Erratum in: J Med Life. 2011 Jan–Mar;4(1):7 p following 123.
14. Hamdoon Z, Jerjes W, Upile T, Hopper C. Optical coherence tomography-guided photodynamic therapy for skin cancer: case study. Photodiagnosis Photodyn Ther. 2011 Mar;8(1):49–52. doi: 10.1016/j.pdpdt.2010.08.004. Epub 2010 Sep 9.
15. Manfredini M, Bettoli V, Sacripanti G et al. The evolution of healthy skin to acne lesions: a longitudinal, in vivo evaluation with reflectance confocal microscopy and optical coherence tomography. J Eur Acad Dermatol Venereol. 2019 Sep;33(9):1768–1774.
16. Manfredini M, Liberati S, Ciardo S et al. Microscopic and functional changes observed with dynamic optical coherence tomography for severe refractory atopic dermatitis treated with dupilumab. Skin Res Technol. 2020 Nov;26(6):779–787.
17. Alex A, Weingast J, Weinigel M et al. Three-dimensional multiphoton/optical coherence tomography for diagnostic applications in dermatology. J Biophotonics. 2013 Apr;6(4):352–62.
18. Lu Q, Jiang G. Progress in the application of reflectance confocal microscopy in dermatology. Postepy Dermatol Alergol. 2021 Oct;38(5):709–715.
19. Nwaneshiudu A, Kuschal C, Sakamoto FH et al. Introduction to confocal microscopy. J Invest Dermatol. 2012 Dec;132(12):e3.
20. Zhao YE, Wu LP, Peng Y, Cheng H. Retrospective analysis of the association between Demodex infestation and rosacea. Arch Dermatol. 2010;146(8):896.
21. Bonnar E, Eustace P, Powell FC. The Demodex mite population in rosacea. J Am Acad Dermatol. 1993;28(3):443.
22. Forton F, Seys B. Density of demodex folliculorum in rosacea: a case-control study using standardized skin-surface biopsy. Br J Dermatol. 1993;128(6):650.
23. Heydenrych I, Kapoor KM, De Boulle K et al. A 10-point plan for avoiding hyaluronic acid dermal filler-related complications during facial aesthetic procedures and algorithms for management. Clin Cosmet Investig Dermatol. 2018; 11: 603–611.
24. Lallas A, Argenziano G, Longo C, et al. Polygonal vessels of rosacea are highlighted by dermoscopy. Int J Dermatol. 2014;53:e325–e327.
25. Rubegni P, Tataranno DR, Nami N, Fimiani M. Rosettes: optical effects and not dermoscopic patterns related to skin neoplasms Australas J Dermatol. 2013;54:271–272.
26. Errichetti E, Stinco G. Dermoscopy in General Dermatology: A Practical Overview. Dermatol Ther (Heidelb). 2016 Dec; 6(4): 471–507.
27. Serarslan G, Makbule Kaya O, Dirican E. Scale and Pustule on Dermoscopy of Rosacea: A Diagnostic Clue for Demodex Species. Dermatol Pract Concept. 2021 Jan 29;11(1):e2021139.
28. Chatterjee M, Shekhar Neema S. Dermatoscopy of Infections and Infestations. Indian Dermatol Online J. 2021 Jan 16;12(1):14–23.
29. Logger JGM, de Vries FMC, van Erp PEJ, et al. Noninvasive objective skin measurement methods for rosacea assessment: a systematic review. Br J Dermatol. 2020 Jan;182(1):55–66.
30. Turgut Erdemir A, Gurel MS, Koku Aksu AE, et al. Demodex mites in acne rosacea: reflectance confocal microscopic study. Australas J Dermatol. 2017;58:e26–e30.
31. Sattler EC, Hoffmann VS, Ruzicka T, et al. Reflectance confocal microscopy for monitoring the density of Demodex mites in patients with rosacea before and after treatment. Br J Dermatol. 2015;173:69–75.
32. Ruini C, Sattler E, Hartmann D, et al. Monitoring structural changes in Demodex mites under topical Ivermectin in rosacea by means of reflectance confocal microscopy: a case series. J Eur Acad Dermatol Venereol. 2017;31:e299–e301.
33. www.who.int/news-room/fact-sheets/detail/herpes-simplex-virus.
34. Narins RS, Jewell M, Rubin M, Cohen J, Strobos J. Clinicalconference: management of rare events following dermal fillers: focal necrosis and angry red bumps. Dermatol Surg. 2006;32:426–434.
35. Dermoscopy in viral infections: An observational study K. M. Sudhakar Rao[1,*], Sakshi S. Gaikwad[1,*] [1]Dept. of Dermatology, Nijalingappa Medical College and HSK Hospital and Research Centre, Navanagar, Bagalkot, Karnataka
36. Cinotti E, Perrot JL, Labeille B et al. Reflectance confocal microscopy for cutaneous infections and infestations. J Eur Acad Dermatol Venereol. 2016 May;30(5):754–63.
37. Lacarrubba F, Verzì AE, Puglisi DF, et al. Line-field confocal optical coherence tomography: a novel, non-invasive

37. imaging technique for a rapid, in-vivo diagnosis of herpes infection of the skin. J Eur Acad Dermatol Venereol. 2021 Jun;35(6):e404–e406.
38. Pathogenesis of acne M Toyoda [1], M Morohashi Department of Dermatology, Faculty of Medicine, Toyama Medical and Pharmaceutical University, 2630 Sugitani, Toyama 930–0194, Japan.
39. Jessop ZM, Welck M, Zinser E et al. Late Presentation of Infected Silicone Granulomas in the Lower Limb. Clin Med Insights Arthritis Musculoskelet Disord. 2018 Feb 22;11:1179544118759020.
40. Manfredini M, Greco M, Farnetani F et al. Acne: morphologic and vascular study of lesions and surrounding skin by means of optical coherence tomography. J Eur Acad Dermatol Venereol. 2017 Sep;31(9):1541–1546.
41. Baran U, Li Y, Choi WJ, Kalkan G, and Wang RK. High Resolution Imaging of Acne Lesion Development and Scarring in Human Facial Skin Using OCT-Based Microangiography. Lasers Surg Med. 2015 Mar;47(3):231–8.
42. M. Manfredini, M. Greco, F. Farnetani, G. Mazzaglia, S. Ciardo, V. Bettoli, A. Virgili and G. Pellacani. In vivo monitoring of topical therapy for acne with reflectance confocal microscopy. Skin Res Technol. 2017 Feb;23(1):36–40.
43. Louise Muguet Guenot L, MD, Morgane Vourc'h Jourdain, MD, Melanie Saint-Jean, MD, Stephane Corvec, MD, PhD, Aurelie Gaultier, MD, Amir Khammari, PhD, Marie Le Moigne, MD, PhD, Aurelie Boisrobert, CRN, Charlotte Paugam, and Brigitte Dreno, MD, PhD. Confocal microscopy in adult women with acne. Int J Dermatol. 2018 Mar;57(3):278–283.
44. Johnson MK. Impetigo. Adv Emerg Nurs J. 2020 Oct/Dec;42(4):262–269.
45. Moormeier DE, Bayles KW. Staphylococcus aureus biofilm: a complex developmental organism. Mol Microbiol. 2017 May;104(3):365–376. Epub 2017 Mar 8.
46. Krzyściak W, Jurczak A, Kościelniak D, Bystrowska B, Skalniak A. The virulence of Streptococcus mutans and the ability to form biofilms.
47. Kuraitis D, Williams L. Decolonization of staphylococcus aureus in healthcare: a dermatology perspective. J Healthc Eng. 2018;2018:1–8.
48. Yi Wang, Valery Leng, Viraj Patel, and K. Scott Phillips. Injections through skin colonized with *Staphylococcus aureus* biofilm introduce contamination despite standard antimicrobial preparation procedures. Sci Rep. 2017 Mar 23;7:45070.
49. Pimenta R, Soares-de-Almeida L, Arzberger E, Ferreira J, Leal-Filipe P, Bastos P M, and Oliveira AL. Reflectance confocal microscopy for the diagnosis of skin infections and infestations. Dermatol Online J. 2020 Mar 15;26(3):13030/qt9qz046f1.
50. Clark GW, Pope SM, Jaboori KA. Diagnosis and treatment of seborrheic dermatitis. Am Fam Physician. 2015 Feb 1;91(3):185–190.
51. Z Zaidi, Z Wahid, R Cochinwala, M Soomro, A Qureishi. Correlation of the density of yeast Malassezia with the clinical severity of seborrhoeic dermatitis. J Pak Med Assoc. 2002 Nov;52(11):504–6.
52. Aneesh Alex, Jessika Weingast, Martin Weinigel, Marcel Kellner-Höfer, Romina Nemecek, Michael Binder, Hubert Pehamberger, Karsten König and Wolfgang Drexler. Three-dimensional multiphoton/optical coherence tomography for diagnostic applications in dermatology. J Biophotonics. 2013 Apr;6(4):352–62.
53. Rajabi-Estarabadi A, Vasquez-Herrera NE, Martinez-Velasco MA et al. Optical coherence tomography in diagnosis of inflammatory scalp disorders. J Eur Acad Dermatol Venereol. 2020 Sep;34(9):2147–2151.
54. Agozzino M, Gonzalez S, Ardigò M. Reflectance Confocal Microscopy for Inflammatory Skin Diseases. Actas Dermosifiliogr. 2016 Oct;107(8):631–9.
55. Agozzino M, Berardesca E, Donadio C et al. Reflectance confocal microscopy features of seborrheic dermatitis for plaque psoriasis differentiation. Dermatology. 2014;229(3):215–21.
56. Ceran C, Aksam E, Demirseren DD et al. Psoriatic Lesions Following Botulinum Toxin: A Injections to the Glabellar Region. J Cutan Aesthet Surg. 2015 Jul-Sep;8(3):178–9.
57. Boone M, Norrenberg S, Jemec G, and Del Marmol V. High-definition optical coherence tomography: adapted algorithmic method for pattern analysis of inflammatory skin diseases: a pilot study. Arch Dermatol Res. 2013; 305(4): 283–297.
58. Simona Laura Ianoşi, Ana Maria Forsea, Mihai Lupu, Mihaela Adriana Ilie, Sabina Zurac, Daniel Boda, Gabriel Ianosi8, Daniela Neagoe, Cristina Tutunaru, Cristina Maria Popa And Constantin Caruntu. Role of modern imaging techniques for the *in vivo* diagnosis of lichen planus (Review). Exp Ther Med. 2019 Feb;17(2):1052–1060.
59. Morsy H, Kamp S, Thrane L, Behrendt N, Saunder B, Zayan H, Elmagid EA, and Jemec GBE. Optical coherence tomography imaging of psoriasis vulgaris: correlation with histology and disease severity. Arch Dermatol Res. 2010 Mar;302(2):105–11.
60. Ella A, Csuka, BS, Suzanne C. Ward, MD, Chloe Ekelem, MD, MPH, David A. Csuka, BS, Marco Ardigò, MD, PhD, and Natasha A. Mesinkovska, MD, PhD. Reflectance Confocal Microscopy, Optical Coherence Tomography, and Multiphoton Microscopy in Inflammatory Skin Disease Diagnosis. Lasers Surg Med. 2021 Aug;53(6):776–797.
61. M. Agozzino, S. Gonzalez, M. Ardigò. Reflectance Confocal Microscopy for Inflammatory Skin Diseases. G Ital Dermatol Venereol. 2015 Oct;150(5):565–73.
62. M Ardigo, C Cota, E Berardesca, S González. Concordance between *in vivo* reflectance confocal microscopy and histology in the evaluation of plaque psoriasis. J Eur Acad Dermatol Venereol. 2009 Jun;23(6):660-7.
63. M Ardigo, M Agozzino, C Longo, A Lallas, V Di Lernia, A Fabiano, A Conti, I Sperduti, G Argenziano, E Berardesca, G Pellacani. Reflectance confocal microscopy for plaque psoriasis therapeutic follow-up during an anti-TNF-α monoclonal antibody: an observational multicenter study. J Eur Acad Dermatol Venereol. 2015 Dec;29(12):2363–8.
64. Wolberink EA, van Erp PE, de Boer-van Huizen RT, van de Kerkhof PC, Gerritsen MJ. Reflectance confocal microscopy: an effective tool for monitoring

ultraviolet B phototherapy in psoriasis. Br J Dermatol. 2012;167:396–403.
65. Y. K. Ba"saran, M. S. Gu€rel, A. T. Erdemir, E. Turan, N. Yurt, and I. S. Bag!ci. Evaluation of the response to treatment of psoriasis vulgaris with reflectance confocal microscopy. Skin Res Technol. 2015 Feb;21(1):18–24.
66. Andrew Creadore, BS, Jacqueline Watchmaker, MD, Mayra B. C. Maymone, DDS, MD, DSc, Leontios Pappas, MD, Neelam A. Vashi, MD, and Christina Lam, MD Boston, Massachusetts. Cosmetic treatment in patients with autoimmune connective tissue diseases. Best practices for patients with lupus erythematosus. J Am Acad Dermatol. 2020 Aug;83(2):343–363.
67. Lafaille P, Benedetto A. Fillers: contraindications, side effects and precautions. J Cutan Aesthet Surg. 2010 Jan–Apr;3(1):16–19.
68. Eastham AB, Liang CA, Femia AN, Lee TC, Vleugels RA, Merola JF. Lupus erythematosus panniculitis-induced facial atrophy: effective treatment with poly-L-lactic acid and hyaluronic acid dermal fillers. J Am Acad Dermatol. 2013;69:e260–e262.
69. A Yazici, H C Er. The correlation of computed tomography in the evaluation of septoplasty patients. Niger J Clin Pract. 2019 Sep;22(9):1196–1200.
70. Wang B, Xu M, Yin N, Wang Y, Song T. Three-Dimensional Computed Tomography Reconstruction and Measurement of Nasal End Deformity in Complete Unilateral Cleft Lip and Palate. Ann Plast Surg. 2021 Nov 1;87(5):562–568.
71. Becker SS, O'Malley BB. Evaluation of sinus computed tomography scans: a collaborative approach between radiology and otolaryngology. Curr Opin Otolaryngol Head Neck Surg. 2013 Feb;21(1):69–73.
72. Jooyeon Kim, Chang Hoi Kim, Jung Ho Oh, Gwan Choi, Jae Hwan Kwon. Saddle Deformity After Septoplasty and Immediate Correction. J Craniofac Surg. 2020 Jan/Feb;31(1):e62–e65.
73. Pravin Mundada, Romain Kohler, Sana Boudabbous, Laurence Toutous Trellu, Alexandra Platon, and Minerva Becker. Injectable facial fillers: imaging features, complications, and diagnostic pitfalls at MRI and PET CT. Insights Imaging. 2017 Dec;8(6):557–572.

CHAPTER 5

Surgical Rhinoplasty

Dario Bertossi, Enrico Robotti, and Carlos Neves

We decided to make a short chapter on an extensive topic to give the reader who is familiar only with non-surgical treatments a brief outline of how a surgical nasal correction differs from the non-surgical approach [1–5]. This will make a clear statement for those who are not surgeons about the differences between a surgical and a non-surgical nasal correction—the posttreatment recovery time, the long-term results, and the possible complications—and we will discuss why sometimes, hopefully rarely, we may have to use a filler injection to give a temporary solution for a necessary postsurgical touch-up. Finally, we will talk about how a non-surgical rhinoplasty may also convince some of our patient population to shift towards a surgical correction to obtain a proper and permanent aesthetic outcome.

Surgical rhinoplasty remains one of the most challenging techniques in plastic surgery and is still one of the most performed facial procedures. The surgical correction of the nose is performed sometimes alone or associated with other facial defect reshaping to achieve a balanced facial result.

Nasal defects can be addressed with different surgical accesses, but the main objective is that whenever a rhinoplasty is done, it must address both nasal function and aesthetics.

Since a normal nasal physiology is a necessary feature, aesthetic goals are primarily dependent on the patient's concerns and expectations. Only an accurate photographic and video documentation during patient consultation can help ensure we and the patients themselves understand the surgical project (see Figure 5.1). This is followed by a very candid discussion of what is and what is not achievable, thus setting realistic expectations for the patient and reducing the risk of postoperative patient dissatisfaction.

Clinical analysis is performed through a set of pictures and a simulation on a desktop computer to illustrate to the patient a possible surgical result. Then an internal analysis with speculum and eventual endoscopic analysis, as well as a cone beam computerized tomography (CBCT), allow us to define the surgical project accurately.

SURGICAL TECHNIQUE

Surgical rhinoplasty is performed almost exclusively under general anesthesia to ensure patient comfort and protection of the airway. However, our surgical maneuvers can result in bleeding, causing secondary complications to upper and lower airways; when the patient is under general anesthesia, we place two nasal swabs (Merocell) deep posteriorly into both upper airways to prevent bleeding into the lower airway areas. We then start with nasal infiltration (see Figure 5.2) before draping to get 10–20 minutes of vasoconstriction through infiltration with cold (4°) 1% lidocaine containing 1:100,000 epinephrine targeting the main vascular network. Using a 27-gauge 13-mm needle, approximately 1 mL of the local solution is injected in the columella base (nasal labial angle area to target columellar arteries) with the same quantity injected along the nasal sidewalls (to target the lateral nasal arteries) and into each nasal base (pyriform aperture). We then proceed with the glabellar area, the nasal dorsum, and the marginal rims of the nose, as well as between the nasal domes. We then inject the internal mucosa of the nasal bones and of the nasal septum. If necessary, the nasal hair within the vestibule is trimmed. The nose is then packed bilaterally with pledges soaked in oxymetazoline. After 10–20 minutes we proceed with the closed-approach transcartilaginous or intracartilaginous incision (see Figure 5.3) or with the open approach, where we make a transcolumellar incision followed by a marginal mucosal incision.

Through these different nasal access routes, we undermine the nasal soft tissues to get to the bony-cartilaginous framework (see Figure 5.4), where during our consultation

SURGICAL RHINOPLASTY

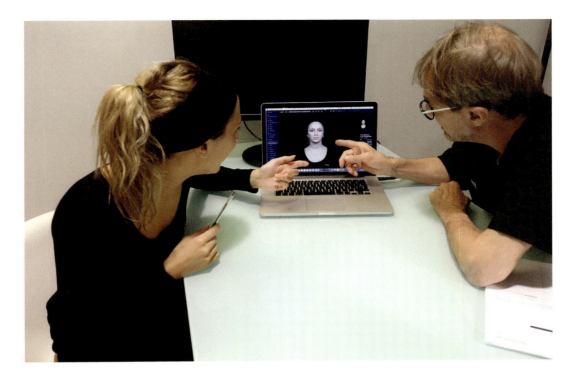

Figure 5.1 Simulation of the possible result with the Adobe Photoshop software.

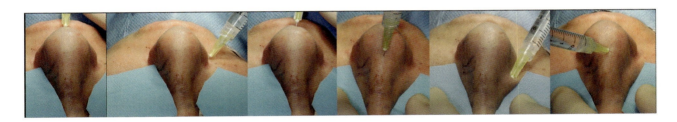

Figure 5.2 The sequence of different points of local anesthesia infiltration during a surgical rhinoplasty.

and surgical plan we have identified the areas to be corrected, whether through cartilaginous incisions and resections or bony rasping. There are also new devices to perform these specific maneuvers through a less traumatic option, such as Piezosurgery (see Figure 5.5) and the Er-Yag laser.

During this operation we may have to choose to reshape the nasal structure for functional or aesthetic purposes, and we can do this by removing some quantity of cartilage and bone or adding one or more cartilaginous grafts (see Figures 5.6 and 5.7) harvested from the nasal area itself, from the ear, or from the rib, which are going to be stabilized with PDS or nylon sutures. These grafts normally are positioned to open the internal nasal

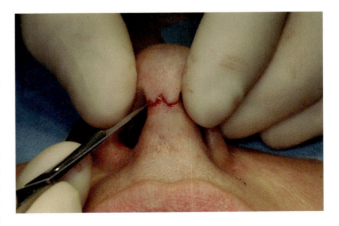

Figure 5.3 After 10–20 minutes we proceed with the open approach. The picture shows a transcolumellar incision followed by a marginal mucosal incision.

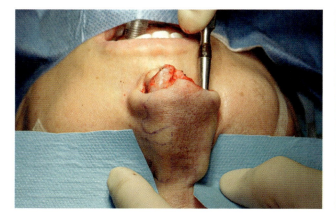

Figure 5.4 Nasal soft tissue undermining.

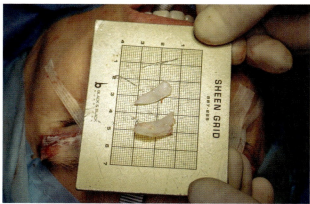

Figure 5.6 Cartilaginous grafts harvested from the nasal septum.

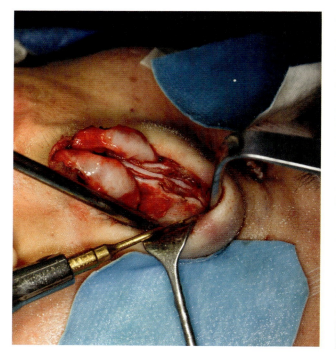

Figure 5.5 Nasal bone osteotomies with the Piezosurgical device.

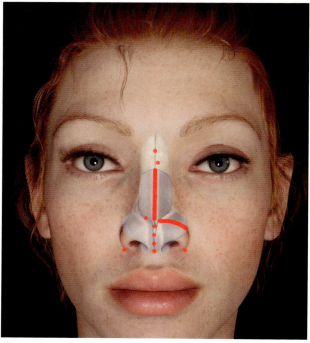

Figure 5.7 Areas of nasal cartilage grafting.

valve area, to correct nasal asymmetries, to give the nasal dorsum or tip support, or finally to achieve nasal finesse.

A more invasive maneuver is osteotomy to narrow the nose, to reduce the bony vault and to close a wide bony vault, and finally to straighten a deviated nasal structure.

Nasal tip refinement sutures or grafts are our last nasal technique for the skin and mucosa (see Figure 5.8). Sometimes skin surgery on the base of the nostril is performed after this final maneuver. We then put Steri-Strips on the nasal skin and a thermoplastic splint onto the Steri-Strips (see Figure 5.9). We control the acute healing phase with small rolls of Surgicell coated with Fucidin ointment that we position into the nostril apices to give support and control infections on

SURGICAL RHINOPLASTY

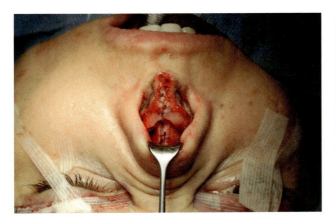

Figure 5.8 Intracartilaginous sutures with PDS 5-0.

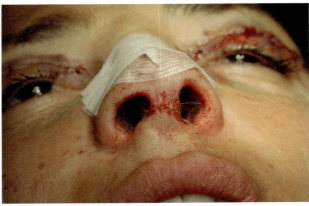

Figure 5.9 Columellar suture.

wound closure. Sutures and Steri-Strips are removed at 7 days, internal splints if positioned are removed after 7 days, and nighttime taping in the supratip area is recommended for 4–6 weeks; alar skin sutures are removed after 10–14 days.

CLINICAL CASE

The patient has a slight nasal hump and right deviation of the nasal septum. The patient was treated with an open approach through a transcolumellar incision, cephalic crus remodeling, nasal hump resection, spreader graft positioning, and diced cartilage positioning. The result shows a harmonious nose with improved brow-tip aesthetic lines (see Figures 5.10–5.13).

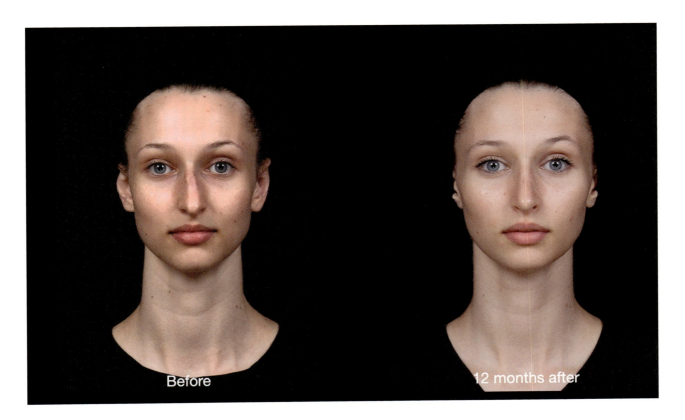

Figure 5.10 Preoperative and postoperative front view of the patient.

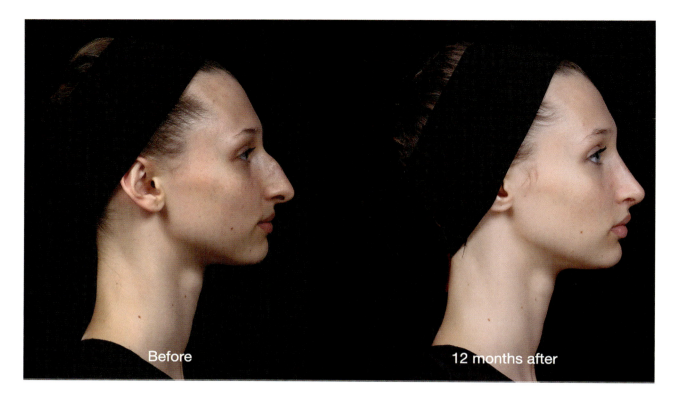

Figure 5.11 Preoperative and postoperative side view of the patient.

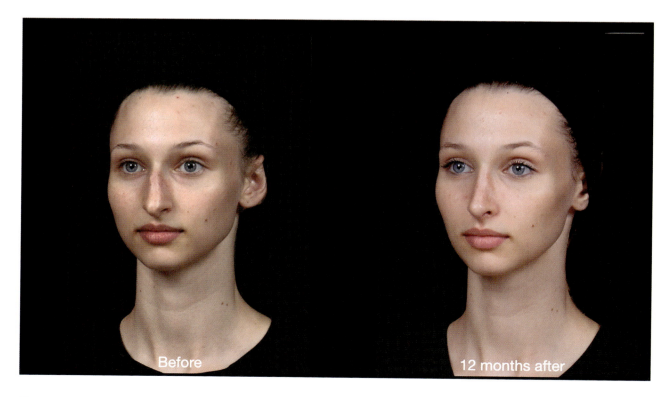

Figure 5.12 Preoperative and postoperative three-quarters view of the patient.

SURGICAL RHINOPLASTY

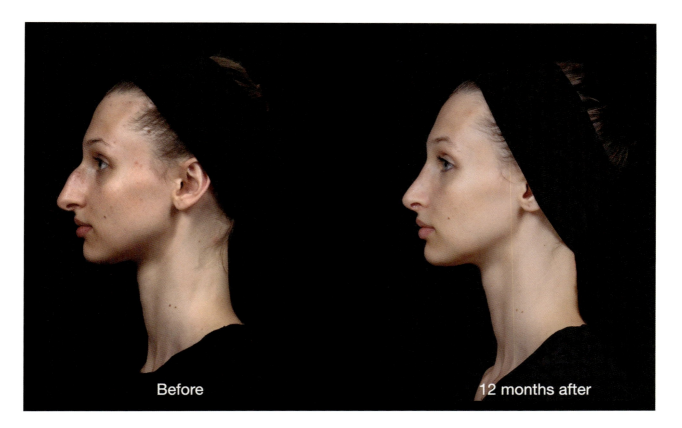

Figure 5.13 Preoperative and postoperative base view of the patient.

CONCLUSIONS

Surgical rhinoplasty relies on accurate visualization of the underlying anatomy to precisely correct anatomical deformities and enhance nasal shape and function. Every facial procedure, surgical and non-surgical, begins with meticulous preoperative analysis of the deformities in conjunction with a clear understanding of the patient's goals. Once realistic expectations are set, thorough preoperative preparation is essential to correct operative execution. Although the level of complexity among rhinoplasty patients is highly variable, the principles and techniques herein are fundamentally comprehensive and will serve as a solid foundation for the rhinoplasty surgeon but will also allow all readers who are not plastic surgeons to understand how different outcomes in terms of defect management can be achieved with this more invasive procedure.

BIBLIOGRAPHY

1. Rohrich RJ, Ahmad J. Rhinoplasty. Plast Reconstr Surg. 2011 Aug;128(2):49e–73e.
2. Ishii LE, Tollefson TT, Basura GJ, et al. Clinical practice guideline: Improving nasal form and function after rhinoplasty. Otolaryngol Head Neck Surg. 2017 Feb;156(2_suppl):S1–S30.
3. Cakmak O, Emre IE, Ozkurt FE. Identifying septal support reconstructions for saddle nose deformity: the Cakmak algorithm. JAMA Facial Plast Surg. 2015 Nov–Dec;17(6):433–439.
4. Ishii LE, Tollefson TT, Basura GJ, et al. Clinical practice guideline: improving nasal form and function after rhinoplasty executive summary. Otolaryngol Head Neck Surg. 2017 Feb;156(2):205–219.
5. Kim DW, Toriumi DM. Management of posttraumatic nasal deformities: the crooked nose and the saddle nose. Facial Plast Surg Clin North Am. 2004 Feb;12(1):111–132.

CHAPTER 6

Non-Surgical Rhinoplasty

Dario Bertossi, Ali Pirayesh, and Alwyn D'Souza

INTRODUCTION

Although the nose has primarily a breathing function, it also represents an aesthetically defining facial feature. Non-surgical rhinoplasty is the term for non-surgical aesthetic improvement with injectable fillers and toxins, whereas surgical nasal reshaping is recognized as rhinoplasty. Rhinoplasty is one of the most requested aesthetic procedures performed by plastic surgeons [1], and for some years now, the American Society for Aesthetic Plastic Surgery and the American Society of Plastic Surgeons have shown a steady increase in requests for non-surgical rhinoplasty [2]; in fact, all the minimally invasive procedures performed in the United States in 2020 accounted for a percentage higher than 85% of all the cosmetic approaches performed that year [3]. The popularity of hyaluronic acid (HA) injection as a well-accepted alternative to surgical rhinoplasty is due to it having immediate aesthetic results, no need for general anesthesia, minimal downtime associated with recovery, cost-effectiveness, a good safety profile [5], and the advantage of being reversible with hyaluronidase [6].

Because of their reversibility, surgeons and physicians consider high-G' HA fillers to be the material with the highest safety for non-surgical rhinoplasty. Nonetheless, it is advisable that this procedure be performed only by highly experienced injectors with an intimate knowledge of injection anatomy and appropriate technique. Patient and product selection, accurate clinical assessment, and correct injection techniques are of critical importance, as the rich vascular network of the nose renders it a high-risk area for severe complications.

Although there are several studies on the longevity and efficacy of various dermal fillers used for various purposes in the facial area [7–11], there are only a few accurate studies focused on the long-term effects of HA fillers in the nasal region [12–15]. Generally, nonsurgical rhinoplasty is considered a non-permanent procedure. Usually, the duration of the effect persists from 8 to 12 months, but based on the authors' experience, it can persist even over 12 months. This could be due to the type of filler used or the individual variability of product degradation.

ETHNIC FEATURES

Nowadays we observe more and more the interchange of races that leads to an ideal of beauty which is more difficult to realize. The growing racial interchange that follows the process we call globalization produces rapid changes in migration patterns, and through social media, the definition of "ethnic" has changed. Our patient requests show that people want to blend in, and their desire is to be a whole with an ethnic group. Ethnicity tends to include race but also depends on culture, nationality, religion, art, music, customs, and history. Therefore, a particular ethnic group includes people with different racial features sharing culture and nationality, depending on sociopolitical patterns, social pressure, or psychological needs.

The anatomy is different in each specific ethnic or racial group, and facial features will vary and will not necessarily coincide with what is found in the specific geographical area where the patient is located. Nasal shape varies dramatically, and noses can be divided into mesorrhine, platyrrhine, and leptorrhine groups. Most patients will have a mixture of these characteristics [6–9].

Platyrrhine Nose

Platyrrhine (flat) noses are found in patients of African descent and Asian groups (see Figure 6.1). They have small nasal bones, a weak and thin nasal septum, a flat shape, and a low radix, and the tip usually lacks support with very acute nasolabial angles. The nostril shape is horizontal with a tendency to flare. The skin is thick.

Mesorrhine Nose

This nose type is between the platyrrhine and the leptorrhine (high) noses (as in mestizo patients of Latin America) (see Figure 6.2). The osseocartilaginous framework is weak (but not as much as in platyrrhine noses) and the skin is thick, the radix is slightly low, and the tip is missing some projection and rotation with more acute nasolabial angles.

Leptorrhine Nose

This nose type belongs to Northern European Caucasian patients with a strong dorsum, high radix, and well-developed nasal bones with a strong middle cartilaginous vault. The skin is thin with an underlying strong osseocartilaginous framework. The tip is defined with adequate projection and rotation because the septal cartilage is more developed, stronger, and thicker than in the other two categories (see Figure 6.3).

NASAL BOUNDARIES

The nose is the center of the face and is surrounded by important anatomical structures and has a profound impact on facial appearance. Even minimal shadowing or asymmetry may be noticed. The upper nasal boundary is the glabella, while the inferior border is the nasal base and inferior nostril border. The ascending process of the upper maxilla defines the lateral borders by an imaginary line between this anatomic structure and the nasal alar attachment. The lateral end of the aesthetic brow forms the tip of a line running from the nasal ala and past the lateral canthus (see Figure 6.4).

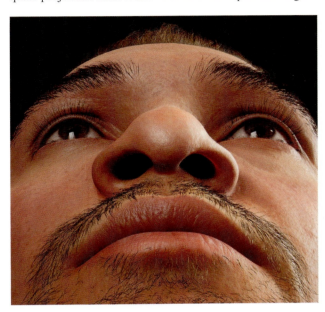

Figure 6.1 Platyrrhine nose.

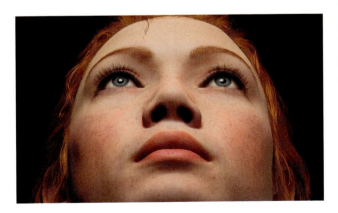

Figure 6.2 Mesorrhine nose.

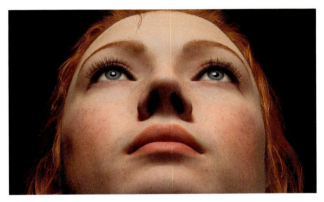

Figure 6.3 Leptorrhine nose.

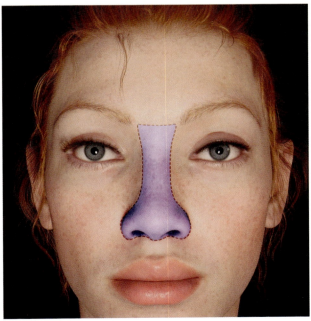

Figure 6.4 Nasal boundaries.

HOW WE DO IT

Patient selection is of utmost importance for nose reshaping with fillers. Both patients with thin and thick skin are suitable candidates for filler rhinomodulation. Patients with thinner skin usually require less product. In these patients, however, any mistake (too much material, either absolutely or relatively) can be visible during and after treatment. As a rule HA should be injected in small quantities for every treated area with constant checkup during injections. Injection volume and skin color should be assessed regularly to avoid any compromise of vascular perfusion. With the aim of taking records, as well as for learning purposes, a nasal grid analysis immediately before filler injection and during treatment (see Figures 6.5 and 6.6) should be traced with standard makeup pencils; analysis allows identification of primary defects—a deep glabella, nasal hump, pseudo hump, double dome or defective nasal projection, nasolabial angle and hidden columella, crooked nose, saddle nose, and nasal base asymmetry.

Nasal botulinum toxin injections are indicated for a sagging nasal tip.

Assessment

Patient age, sex, and nasal defects are recorded for all enrolled patients at baseline. Follow-up clinical examinations are carried out at 12 hours, 1 day, 7–10 days, 30 days, and 10 months. The first posttreatment evaluation for efficacy and eventual touch-up is to be conducted at week 4.

All patients are subjected to an accurate photogrammetric analysis. Photographs are taken before the injection

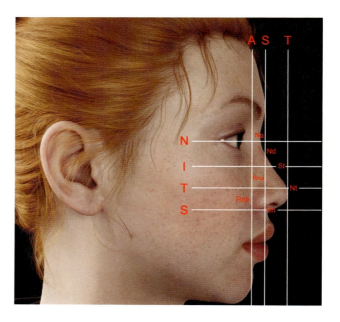

Figure 6.6 Nasal grid.

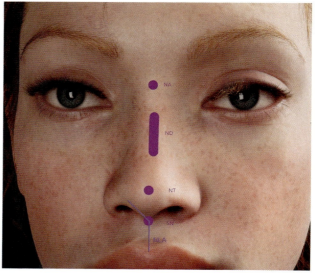

Figure 6.7 Significant nasal points to be treated with filler.

and at follow-up intervals, in frontal, lateral, 45 degrees bilateral, basal, superior, and above and below views (see Chapter 3). We evaluate the volume stability with ultrasound and clinical pictures.

Taking as a reference the mid-pupillary line (MPL), we monitor the sagittal pre- and posttreatment distance of the following soft-tissue points: nasion (Na), nasal dorsum (Nd), nasal tip (Nt), subnasal (Sn), and nasolabial angle (NLA). All these anthropometric factors are measured and compared before and after treatment (see Figure 6.7).

Complications must also be recorded and reported to the manufacturing company and assessed throughout treatment and follow-up.

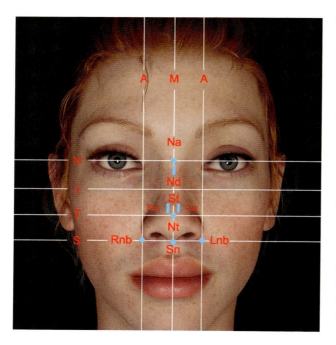

Figure 6.5 Nasal grid.

Nasal Base Retrusion

EFFECT OF INJECTION: Pushes up the nasal base, reduces the depth of the nasal-labial fold
SURGICAL ALIAS: Pyriform aperture graft (see Figure 6.8)
Area: Inject on the base of the nose at the pyriform aperture area (see Figure 6.9a). A slow, supraperiosteal injection should be performed.
Defect: Retrusion of the upper maxilla
Device: Needle 27G
Position: Deep to the bone perpendicular to it (see Figure 6.9b)
Filler type: High or very high G'
Amount: Between 0.2 and 0.5 mL per side

Hidden Columella Nasal Base Retrusion (See Figure 6.10a)

EFFECT OF INJECTION: Pushes out the mid-columellar area, opens the nasal-labial angle
SURGICAL ALIAS: Septal extended graft, caudal portion of the shield graft (see Figure 6.10b).
Area: Inject in the middle point of the columella, holding the columella between the index and the thumb. A slow, intradermal injection should be performed (Figure 6.11a).
Defect: Flat columella
Device: Needle 27G
Position: Deep dermis (see Figure 6.11b)
Filler type: High or very high G'
Amount: Between 0.1 and 0.2 mL

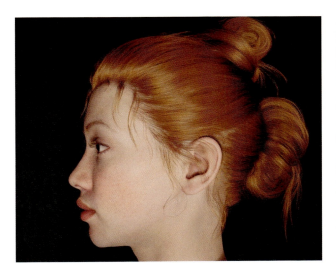

Figure 6.8a Nasal base retrusion defect.

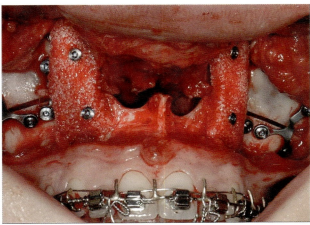

Figure 6.8b Nasal base retrusion defect treated surgically with customized Medpore grafts.

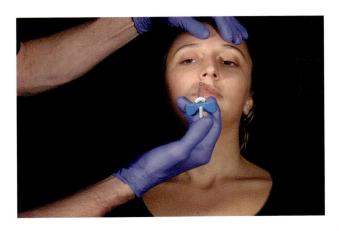

Figure 6.9a Nasal base retrusion defect treated with filler: Position of the needle on the patient.

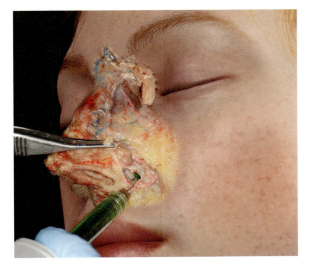

Figure 6.9b Nasal base retrusion defect treated with filler: Position of the needle on the cadaver—bone of the pyriform aperture.

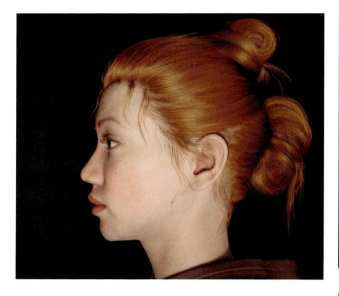

Figure 6.10a Hidden columella defect.

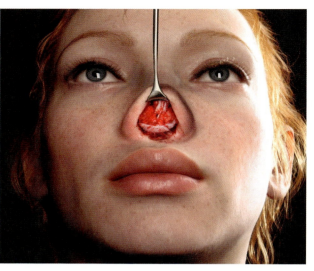

Figure 6.10b Hidden columella defect treated surgically with customized infratip cartilage grafts.

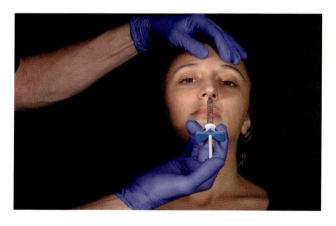

Figure 6.11a Hidden columella defect treated with filler: Position of the needle on the patient.

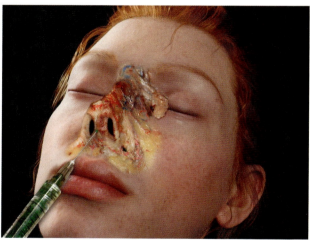

Figure 6.11b Hidden columella defect treated with filler: Position of the needle on the cadaver—superficial fat area (deep dermis).

Closed Nasal Labial Angle Nasal Base Retrusion (See Figure 6.12a)

EFFECT OF INJECTION: Pushes up the columellar base, opens the nasal-labial angle

SURGICAL ALIAS: Anterior nasal spine graft (see Figure 6.12b)

Area: Inject in the middle point of the nasal-labial angle, holding the columellar base between the index and the thumb. Age-related columellar retraction because of maxillary resorption and soft tissue change gives the illusion of tip caudal rotation or droop. A slow, supraperiosteal injection should be performed (Figure 6.13a).

Defect: Closed nasal-labial angle
Device: Needle 27G
Position: Deep to the bone (see Figure 6.13b)
Filler type: High or very high G'
Amount: Between 0.2 and 0.5 mL

Dependent Tip: Tip Injection (See Figure 6.14a)

EFFECT OF INJECTION: Pushes out the tip area between the domes, gives the nose projection. To be associated with the ANS injection and columellar injection.

SURGICAL ALIAS: Septal extension graft (see Figure 6.14b).

Area: Inject in the middle point of the tip between the domes holding the tip between the index and the thumb. A slow, intradomal injection should be performed.

Defect: Dependent tip
Device: Needle 27G
Position: Deep between the domes (see Figure 6.15)
Filler type: High or very high G'
Amount: Between 0.1 and 0.5 mL

NON-SURGICAL RHINOPLASTY

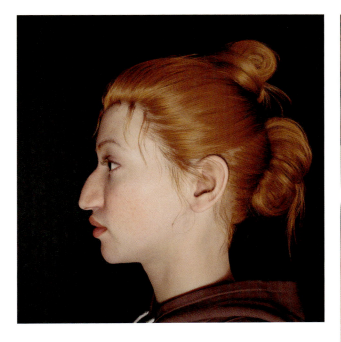

Figure 6.12a Closed nasal-labial angle defect.

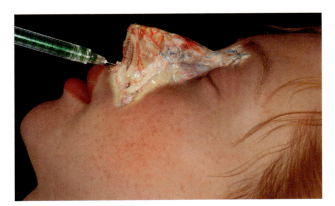

Figure 6.13a Closed nasal-labial angle defect treated with filler: position of the needle on the patient.

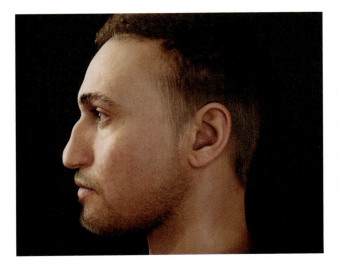

Figure 6.14a Dependent tip defect.

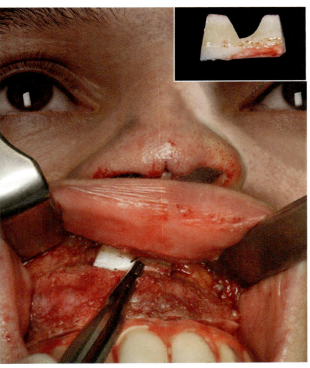

Figure 6.12b Closed nasal-labial angle defect surgical correction with a rib cartilage graft.

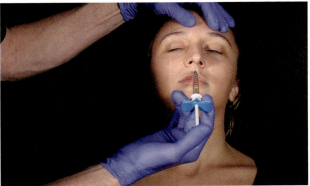

Figure 6.13b Closed nasal-labial angle defect treated with filler: Position of the needle on the cadaver—deep to the bone (anterior nasal spine).

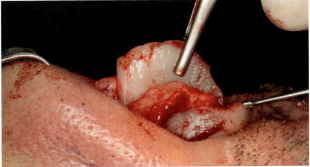

Figure 6.14b Dependent tip defect treated surgically with customized septal extension cartilage graft.

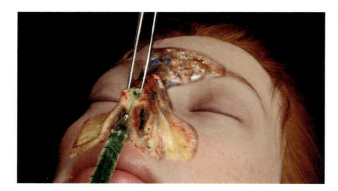

Figure 6.15 Dependent tip defect treated with filler: Position of the needle on the cadaver—deep between cartilaginous domes (apical portion of the alar cartilages, which creates an arch between medial and lateral cruras).

Nasal Hump (See Figure 6.16a)

EFFECT OF INJECTION: Pushes up the nasal dorsum below and above the nasal hump. To be associated with the nasal tip and nasal dorsum injection.
SURGICAL ALIAS: Dorsal resection or associated with a glabellar graft (see Figure 6.16b).

Area: Inject in the middle point of the tip between the domes, then the glabella (Figure 6.17a and b) and then the nasal dorsum. A slow, supraperiosteal and supraperichondral injection should be performed.

Defect: Various degrees of nasal hump

Device: Needle 27G or cannula 38 mm 25G

Position: Deep between the domes, deep to the bone in the glabella, deep to the bone in the nasal dorsum (see Figure 6.17c and d)

Filler type: High or very high G'

Amount: Between 0.1 and 1 mL

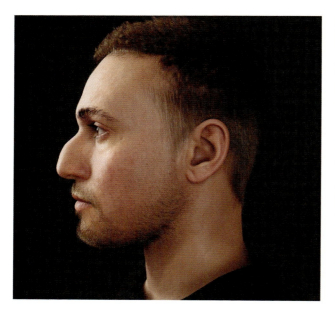

Figure 6.16a Nasal hump defect.

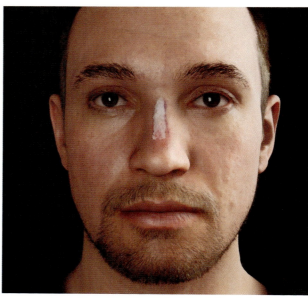

Figure 6.16b Nasal hump defect treated surgically with customized cartilage graft.

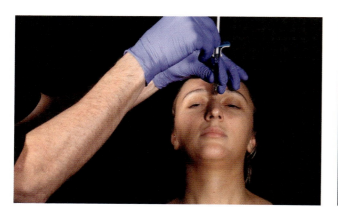

Figure 6.17a Nasal hump defect treated with filler: Position of the needle on the patient.

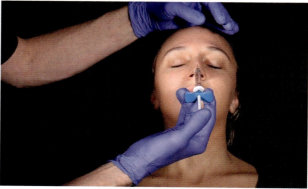

Figure 6.17b Nasal hump defect treated with filler: Position of the needle on the patient.

NON-SURGICAL RHINOPLASTY

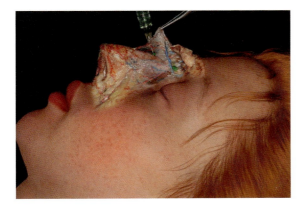

Figure 6.17c Nasal hump defect treated with filler: Position of the needle on the cadaver—deep to the bone with the needle.

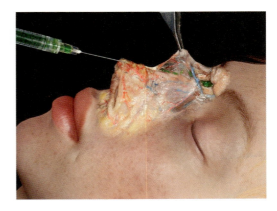

Figure 6.17d Nasal hump defect treated with filler: Position of the cannula on the cadaver—deep to the bone and cartilage.

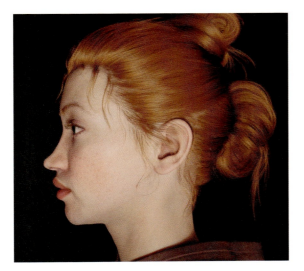

Figure 6.18a Saddle nose defect.

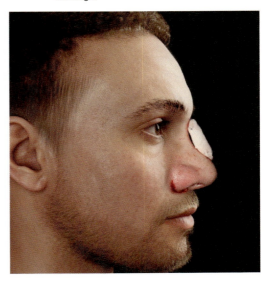

Figure 6.18b Saddle nose defect treated surgically with diced cartilage graft into a collagen membrane.

Saddle Nose (See Figure 6.18a)

EFFECT OF INJECTION: Pushes up the columellar base, opens the nasal-labial angle

SURGICAL ALIAS: Nasal dorsum graft (see Figure 6.18b)

Area: Inject in the middle point of the tip between the domes, then the glabella, then the nasal dorsum. If the sagittal dorsal defect is more than 3 mm, the dorsum correction should be achieved over multiple sessions. A slow, supra-periosteal, and subdermal injection should be performed.

Defect: Various degrees of nasal void

Device: Needle 27G or cannula 38 mm 25G

Position: Deep between the domes, deep to the bone in the glabella and deep to the bone in the nasal dorsum (see Figure 6.19)

Filler type: High or very high G'

Amount: Between 0.1 and 1 mL

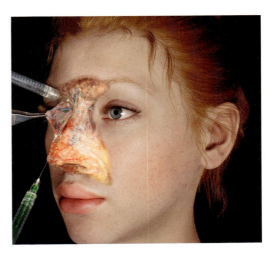

Figure 6.19 Saddle nose defect treated with filler: Position of the cannula on the cadaver—deep to the bone and cartilage.

Overprojected Nose (See Figure 6.20a)

EFFECT OF INJECTION: Fills the nasal dorsum, the nasal base, and the malar area, as well as the infraorbital area
SURGICAL ALIAS: Pyriform aperture graft and malar graft (see Figure 6.20b)
Area: Inject in the middle point of the tip between the domes, then the glabella, then the nasal dorsum. If the sagittal dorsal defect is more than 3 mm, the dorsum correction should be achieved over multiple sessions. Inject also the nasal-labial area, cheek area, and upper lip area. A slow, supraperiosteal and subdermal injection should be performed.
Defect: Various degrees of nasal overprojection
Device: Needle 27G or cannula 38 mm 25G
Position: Deep between the domes, deep to the bone in the glabella, and deep to the bone in the nasal dorsum (see Figure 6.21).
Filler type: High or very high G'
Amount: Between 0.1 and 1 mL

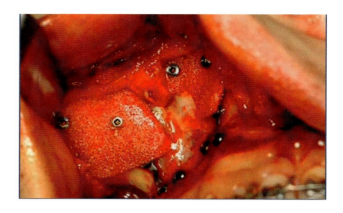

Figure 6.20b Overprojected nose defect treated surgically with customized malar and infraorbital Medpore grafts.

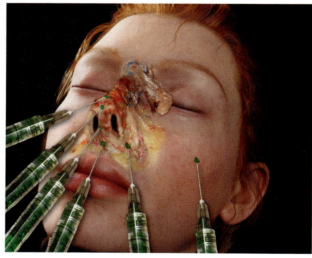

Figure 6.21 Overprojected nose defect treated with filler: Position of the needle on the cadaver—deep between the domes, deep on the bone on the glabella and the nasal dorsum, deep to the bone in the malar and infraorbital region.

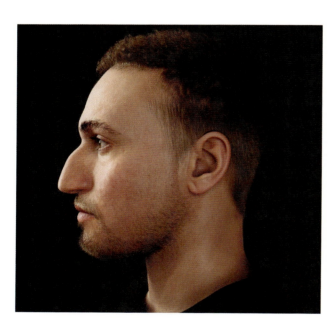

Figure 6.20a Overprojected nose defect.

Deep Glabella (See Figure 6.22a)

EFFECT OF INJECTION: Pushes out the glabella
SURGICAL ALIAS: Glabellar graft (see Figure 6.22b).
Area: Inject in the middle point of the nasion, holding the glabella between the index and the thumb. A slow, intradomal injection should be performed.
Defect: Various degrees of glabellar defects.
Device: Needle 27G or cannula 38 mm 25G
Position: Deep between the domes, deep to the bone in the glabella, and deep to the bone in the nasal dorsum (see Figure 6.23)
Filler type: High or very high G'
Amount: Between 0.2 and 0.6 mL

NON-SURGICAL RHINOPLASTY

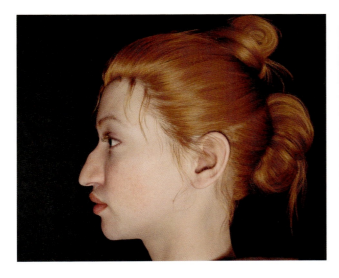

Figure 6.22a Deep glabella defect.

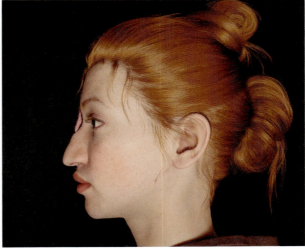

Figure 6.22b Deep glabella defect treated surgically with customized cartilage graft.

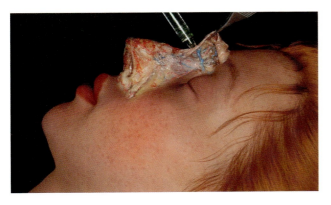

Figure 6.23 Deep glabella treated with filler: Position of the needle on the cadaver—deep on the bone on the glabella and the nasal dorsum.

Deviated Nose (See Figure 6.24a)

EFFECT OF INJECTION: Corrects asymmetries
SURGICAL ALIAS: Spreader or batten, various grafts (see Figure 6.24b)
Area: Inject in the middle point of the nasal dorsum and massage gently to distribute the filler
Defect: Various degrees of nasal deviations
Device: Needle 27G or cannula 38 mm 25G
Position: Deep to the bone and over the cartilage (see Figure 6.25a and b)
Filler type: High or very high G'
Amount: Between 0.2 and 1 mL

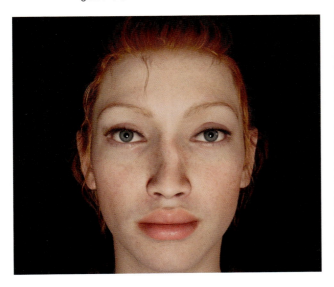

Figure 6.24a Deviated nose defect.

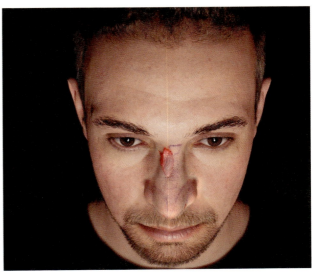

Figure 6.24b Deviated nose defect treated surgically with customized cartilage overlay graft.

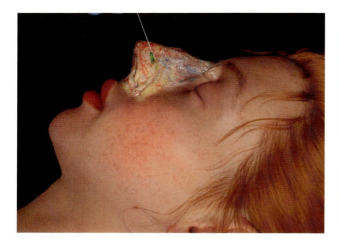
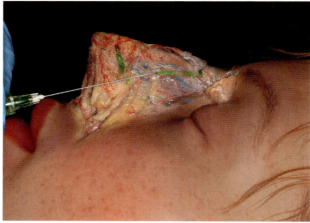

Figure 6.25a-b Deviated nose defect treated with filler: Position of the needle on the cadaver—deep on the bone and on the cartilage.

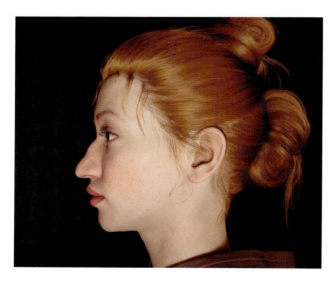

Figure 6.26 Secondary nose defect.

Secondary Defects (See Figure 6.26)

Non-surgical rhinoplasty in patients who have undergone previous rhinoplasty can increase the risk of vascular compromise. In secondary rhinoplasty patients, it is mandatory to inject HA slowly to avoid whitening of the skin.

Crooked Nose Deformity (See Figure 6.27)

With a crooked nose deformity, the goal is to fill the shadows. To avoid the lateral nasal artery, the needle must enter on the midline. Once we have reached the periosteum or perichondrium, we must slide laterally deep to the defect or inject medially and mold laterally. The injection sequence is as follows: Sn, Rnb or Lnb, Nt, Na, Nd, and St.

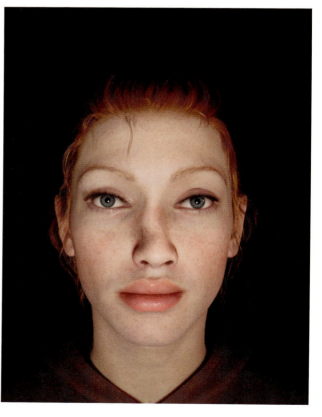

Figure 6.27 Crooked nose defect.

NON-SURGICAL RHINOPLASTY

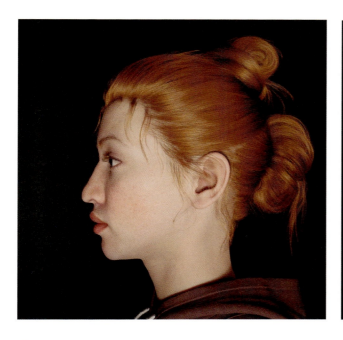

Figure 6.28a Nasal alar retraction or collapse.

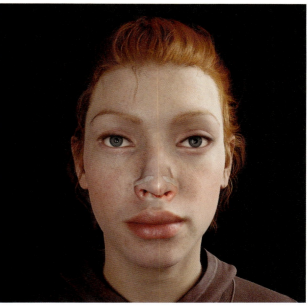

Figure 6.28b Nasal alar retraction or collapse treated surgically with customized cartilage alar rim graft.

Alar Retraction or Collapse (See Figure 6.28a)

EFFECT OF INJECTION: Corrects the asymmetries
SURGICAL ALIAS: Alar rim graft (see Figure 6.28b)
Alar retraction or collapse can be reshaped with the Rna and Lna injection. This technique is for expert injectors, which means that nasal surgeons or injectors should have more than 2 years of experience in full facial rejuvenation because of the high risk of skin necrosis. Filling is performed in the deep subdermal layer, in small volumes under low pressure, close to the rim; injection must cease if blanching is noted.
Area: Inject in the alar border and massage gently to distribute the filler
Defect: Various degrees of nasal deviations
Device: Needle 27G or cannula 38 mm 25G
Position: Subcutaneous (see Figure 6.29).
Filler type: High or very high G'
Amount: Between 0.01 and 0.1 mL

Injection Plan and Procedure

The procedure begins with skin disinfection using a 75% alcohol solution. The nasal grid analysis is traced, and the treatment performed by a sole injector following the injecting protocol. Following the nasal grid points, associated defects of the nasal structure are treated in this sequence: Sn, Rnb and Lnb, Nt, and Na and Nd. The remaining points through the grid are right and left nasal ala and right and left nasal base (Rna, Lna and Rnb, Lnb) for each side.

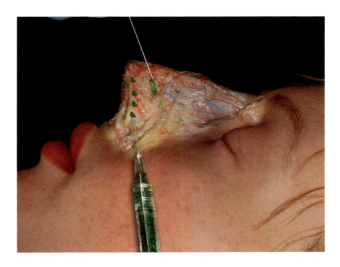

Figure 6.29 Nasal alar retraction or collapse treated with filler: Position of the filler on the cadaver—subcutaneous.

We use an HA gel with a very high G' (VYC-25; Allergan, Inc., Irvine, Calif.), 25 mg/mL with 0.3% lidocaine, characterized by intrinsic viscosity and cohesivity. We use a 27-gauge, 13-mm needle, injecting through multiple entry points or a 38-mm 25G cannula with a single or double entry point. The **volume range** of the HA filler injected is between 0.4 and 1.8 mL.

Key points:

1. **SKIN DISINFECTION**: Using a 75% alcohol solution.
2. **MATERIAL**: Inject a high G' HA (20–25 mg/mL).

3. **DEVICE**: Use 27G 13-mm needle or 25G 38-mm cannula. Only expert injectors can use fillers with different devices (HA transfer in insulin syringes or use of smaller-diameter needles for more superficial injections or use of motorized devices).
4. **INJECTION LOCATION**: This depends on the area to be injected. It is well documented that the major branches of arteries and veins, generally speaking, lie away from the midline [9,10]. This is not valid for noses treated with rhinoplasty where surgical undermining has distorted the normal anatomy. Differences in the anatomy profile and setting might put patients at higher risk for a discouraging intravascular injection. It is recommended to always aspirate for 5–7 seconds before injection with small volumes, with constant patient monitoring mandatory for signs of vascular compromise. The surgeon should pinch the soft tissue in the midline. Actually, the area of treatment is often pinched up and even compressed throughout the injection procedure in order to prevent a side displacement of HA. Side or lateral defects, where there may be an enhanced risk of an erroneously mediated intravascular injection, could be most likely corrected, in a safe way, by selecting a midline injection, then followed by molding HA and properly displacing laterally with respect to the body. This approach is crucial where lateral defects to be corrected are present and should allow prevention of an enhanced risk of intravascular injection by leaving the midline.

The sequence is:
   a) Subnasal or anterior nasal spine (Sn): 27G 13-mm needle, inject midline deep to the bone (see Figure 6.30)
   b) Right and left nasal base or pyriform aperture (Rnb and Lnb): 27G 13-mm needle, inject deep to the bone (see Figure 6.31)
   c) Nasal tip or the area between the domes (Nt): 27G 13-mm needle, inject midline, deep to the subcutaneous layer in the areolar tissue that joins the domes; we can also make an entry point with the 38-mm 25G cannula in the infratip area (see Figure 6.32)
   d) Nasion or the area above the glabella (Na): 27G 13-mm needle, inject midline, deep to the bone; we can also make an entry point with the 38-mm 25G cannula in the infratip area (see Figure 6.33)
   e) Nasal dorsum (Nd): 27G 13-mm needle, inject midline, deep to the bone; we can also make an entry point with the 38-mm 25G cannula in the infratip area (see Figure 6.34)
   f) Supratip in the boundary between the nasal septum and the domes (st): 27G 13-mm needle, inject midline, deep to the bone; we can also make an entry point with the 38-mm 25G cannula in the infratip area (see Figure 6.35)
   g) Infratip or midcolumellar area (it): 27G 13-mm needle, inject midline, deep to the bone; we can also make an entry point with the 38-mm 25G cannula in the infratip area (see Figure 6.36)

After the treatment the patients are asked to avoid unnecessary external compression of the nose (from wearing heavy eyeglasses or hard massage), which could cause filler displacement, indentation, or depression of the dorsal surface.

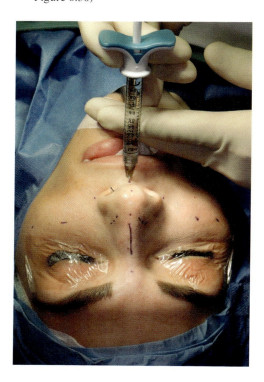

Figure 6.30 Anterior nasal spine injection.

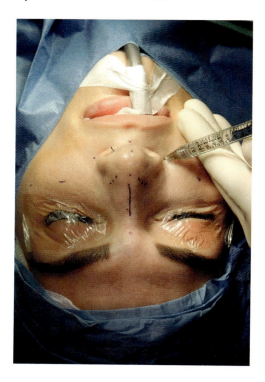

Figure 6.31 Right nasal base injection.

NON-SURGICAL RHINOPLASTY

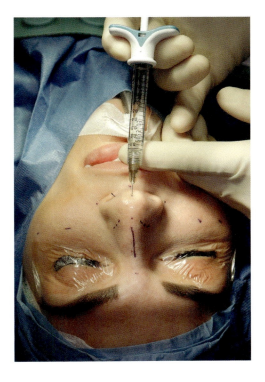

Figure 6.32 Interdomal injection.

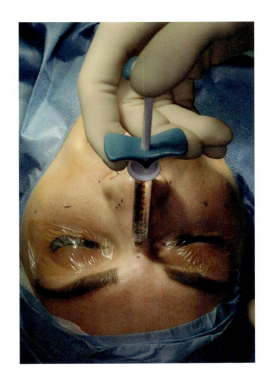

Figure 6.33 Glabellar injection.

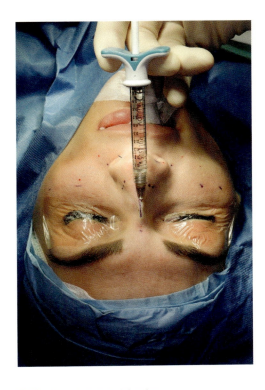

Figure 6.34 Nasal dorsum injection.

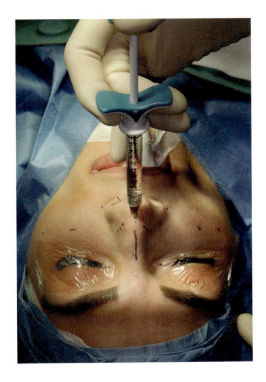

Figure 6.35 Supratip area injection.

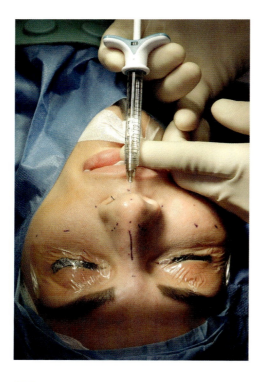

Figure 6.36 Infratip lobule injection.

5) **AMOUNT OF HA**: We provide the amount of HA at the very first session.

- Subnasale or anterior nasal spine (Sn): Between 0.1 and 0.5 mL of HA
- Right and left nasal base or pyriform aperture (Rnb and Lnb): Between 0.2 and 0.5 mL of HA
- Nasal tip or the area between the domes (Nt): Between 0.1 and 0.3 mL of HA
- Nasion or the area above the glabella (Na): Between 0.1 and 0.4 mL of HA
- Nasal dorsum (Nd): Between 0.1 and 0.8 mL of HA
- Supratip in the boundary between the nasal septum and the domes (st): Between 0.1 and 0.25 mL of F HA
- Infratip or midcolumellar area (it): Between 0.1 and 0.4 mL of HA

HOW I DO IT: BOTULINUM TOXINS

Bunny Lines

Bunny lines are made by the transverse portion of the nasalis muscle alongside with the levator labii superioris alaeque nasi muscle. The dose per injection site is 2 U per side in both male and female individuals. The injection is performed at a 45-degree angle to the skin with a low-to-high direction. Usually, the physician performs one single injection on either side of the nose, in the middle of the targeted region. The entry side of the needle is restricted to the tip solely, because the muscle is quite close underneath the skin plane. Care should be taken to not inject too much laterally, to avoid functional interference with the levator labii superioris alaeque nasi muscle, which might produce an undesirable elongation of the upper lip. Very often, once treating the bunny lines, procerus muscle treatment is carried out concurrently in order to address the horizontal lines at the nasal root.

Sagging Nasal Tip

The target muscle used for treating a sagging nose tip is the depressor septi nasi. In case of hypertonicity, the so-called depressor septi nasi shifts on a lower plane than the nose tip, which then is more visible when the subject smiles or laughs. In order to treat a sagging nasal tip, surgeons recommend a single injection with a 2–4 U dose in both female and male patients. Treatment is performed by inserting one-quarter of a 30G needle at the base of the columella, pointing toward the nasal spine. The treatment causes the upward rotation of the nose tip. The assessment of clinical hallmarks could be a crucial step for the right selection of patients, as any treatment of the sagging nose tip should be rejected in individuals with a long upper lip. A long caudal septum represents also a counterindication to toxin treatment, as it prevents the requested tip rotation.

Statistical Analysis on Treated Patients and Stability of Filler

Descriptive statistics are provided throughout, including mean, standard deviation, and range for continuous variables and frequency and percentage for categorical variables.

Results

A total of 1,000 patients were included in the analysis. The mean age was 36 ± 7 years (range, 19–57 years). The group included 169 males (30.8%) and 831 females (69.2%). Patients were followed up for 14 months.

The nasal grid became the reference for the quantity and sequencing of injections, increasing the potential for reproducible future treatment. The following defects were recorded and treated at baseline utilizing the grid (Table 6.1): dorsal nasal hump, n = 821 (83.2%); deprojected nose, n = 788 (10.3%); tip downrotated, n = 211 (6.5%). No more nose treatments were done on patients during the follow-up period.

The average injection volume was 1.0 ± 0.5 mL for nasal dorsum augmentation, 1.0 ± 0.4 mL for tip rotation, and

Table 6.1 Defects Identified and Treated

	Dorsal Hump	Deprojected Nose	Downrotated Tip
Total (n = 1000)	821	788	211
Female (n = 831)	568	545	146
Male (n = 169)	253	243	65

1.7 ± 0.6 mL for whole nose augmentation. By specific subsites of injection, the average injected volume was 0.4 ± 0.3 mL for the glabella-to-radix area, 0.9 ± 0.5 mL for the nasal dorsum, 0.5 ± 0.3 mL for the nasal tip, and 0.6 ± 0.4 mL for the columella-nasolabial junction.

We focused especially on morphological changes in the long term through an accurate photogrammetric analysis and the execution of a nasal ultrasound in selected patients. At the control 14 months after treatment, all patients were re-evaluated.

POSTTREATMENT

The patient should be furnished with written posttreatment instructions and contact numbers. Commonsense advice such as washing the face with uncontaminated water, using a new lipstick, and applying uncontaminated facial products should be given. Patients must avoid sun exposure for 1 week and the sauna or intense exercises for 72 hours.

- The injector/clinic should be available by phone for 48 hours postprocedure.
- It is good practice to have a staff member call the patient the next day.

Non-surgical rhinoplasty is one of the newest applications of dermal fillers to improve the profile and to correct defects of the nose and is becoming the gold standard in nasal aesthetics, as it is a safe and predictable technique with a significant degree of customer satisfaction [16].

The careful and proper selection of eligible patients, with correct knowledge of nasal anatomy and of filler rheology, are crucial [4]. The most common indications are minor defects of the nose, such as a pronounced hump, underprojected tip, nasal depressions, saddle nose, and corrections of trauma outcomes. Moreover, the injection of HA filler can also be used as a complement to surgery or for the correction of minor postsurgical defects (5–15% of surgical rhinoplasties) [6]. However, if a patient's expectations are greater than is possible with HA injections, it is necessary to turn to rhinoplasty.

A high degree of patient satisfaction is explained by the immediate aesthetic results that can be obtained with fillers, the stable results, no need for general anesthesia, and low cost. The non-permanent nature of HA and reversibility with hyaluronidase are also favorable properties for fillers [17]. In addition to these benefits, a key factor for many patients is the absence of recovery time; non-surgical rhinoplasty with an HA filler allows individuals to return to work and other commitments as rapidly as the same day [18–34].

Other types of semi-permanent dermal fillers are also available, but semi-permanent fillers such as calcium HA or permanent soft tissue fillers can also move and produce severe granulomatous reactions, with nasal cellulitis, nodules, and ulcers that are difficult to treat and cannot be reversed in the case of intravascular injection [22,23]. For this reason, nowadays they are almost never used in aesthetic medicine.

Generally, due to the gradual reabsorption of the filler, results last up to 8–12 months after treatment, making it a valid minimally invasive alternative to surgical rhinoplasty. Consequently, to maintain the effects, it is necessary to repeat the treatment once a year.

Limitations of Non-Surgical Rhinoplasty

We suggest avoiding this technique in overprojected noses, posttraumatic noses, nose defects secondary to cleft lip, overinjected noses, noses previously injected with permanent or semi-permanent fillers, noses treated with alloplastic grafts, Wegener's defects, saddle noses caused by cocaine abuse, reconstructed noses, and noses injected in a poor sterile environment.

CLINICAL CASES

Patient 1: This was a female patient with nasal dorsum irregularities and associated microgenia. We injected 2 mL of very high G' filler on the nasal base (0.4 per side), anterior nasal spine (0.3 mL), nasal tip (0.1 mL), supratip area (0.15 mL), glabella (0.2 mL), and nasal dorsum (0.35 mL). We then performed a 1.2-mL injection on the midpoint of the chin, 0.9 mL on the lowest point of the chin bone, and 0.2 mL on the pogonion. We can appreciate the results before and after on the front (Figure 1), profile (Figure 2), and three-quarters view (Figure 3). The patient was satisfied with a good long-term result at 1 year postinjection.

Patient 2: This was a female patient with nasal dorsum irregularities and associated upper lip deficiency. We injected 1.4 mL of very high G' filler on the nasal base (0.3 per side), anterior nasal spine (0.3 mL), nasal tip (0.1 mL), supratip area (0.1 mL), glabella (0.2 mL), and nasal dorsum (0.3 mL). We then performed a 10-mL injection on the upper lip, distributing the injections first on the lower lip vermilion body, then on the vermilion body of the upper lip, and finally defining the vermilion border. We can appreciate the results before and after on the front (Patient 1 Figure 1), profile (Patient 1 Figure 2), and three-quarters view (Patient 1 Figure 3). The patient was satisfied with a good long-term result at 1.4 years postinjection.

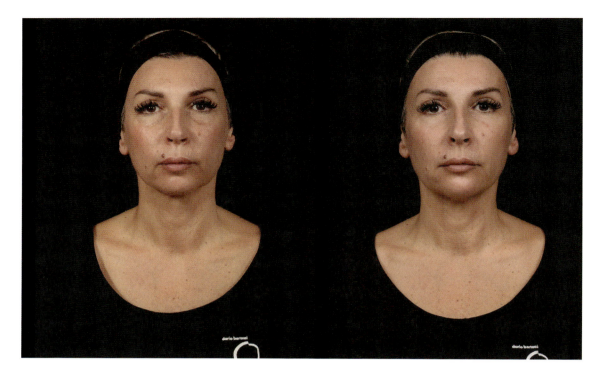

Patient 1 Figure 1 Front view of a female patient with asymmetric brow-tip esthetic lines and microgenia: Improvement of the brow-tip aesthetic lines and chin projection.

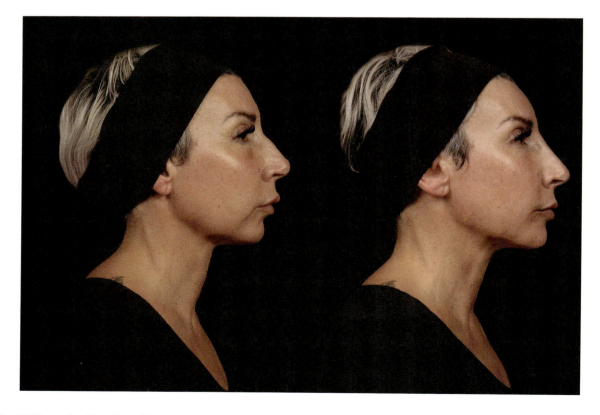

Patient 1 Figure 2 Side view of the female patient.

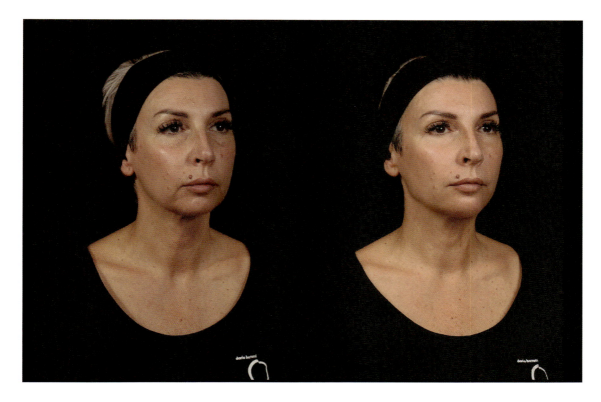

Patient 1 Figure 3 Three-quarters view of the female patient.

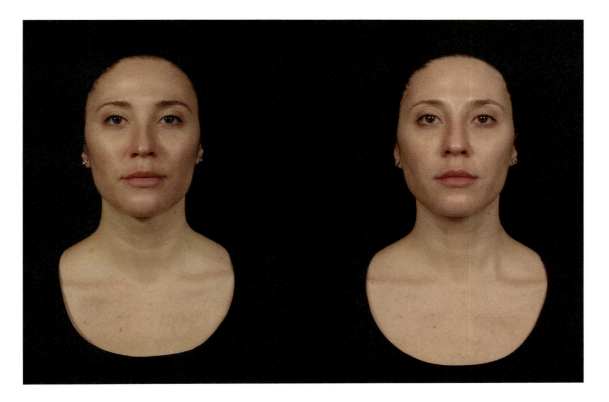

Patient 2 Figure 1 Front view of a female patient with asymmetric brow-tip aesthetic lines with convergence on the nasal dorsum: Improvement of the brow-tip aesthetic lines and nasal-labial angle.

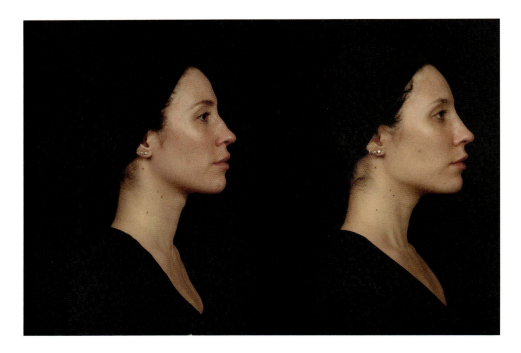

Patient 2 Figure 2 Side view of the female patient.

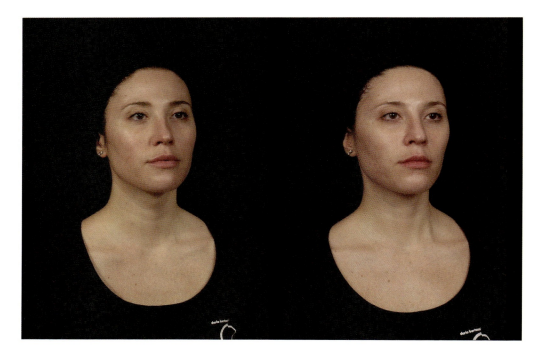

Patient 2 Figure 3 Three-quarters view of the female patient.

Patient 3: This was a female patient with a slight nasal dorsum hump and associated microgenia. We injected 2 mL of very high G' filler on the nasal base (0.4 per side), anterior nasal spine (0.3 mL), nasal tip (0.1 mL), supratip area (0.15 m:), glabella (0.2 mL), and nasal dorsum (0.35 mL). We then performed a 1.2-mL injection on the midpoint of the chin, 0.9 mL on the lowest point of the chin bone, and 0.2 mL on the pogonion. We can appreciate the results before and after on the front (Figure 1), profile (Figure 2), and three-quarters view (Figure 3). The patient was satisfied with a good long-term result at 1 year postinjection.

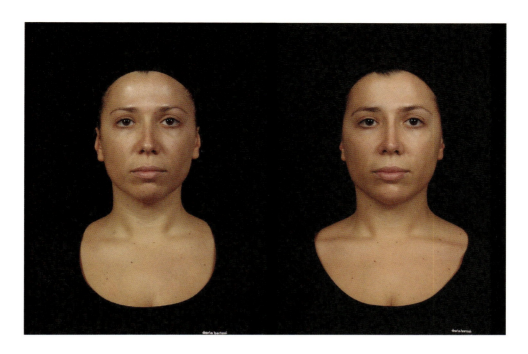

Patient 3 Figure 1 Front view of a female patient with asymmetric brow-tip esthetic lines and microgenia: Improvement of the brow-tip esthetic lines and chin projection.

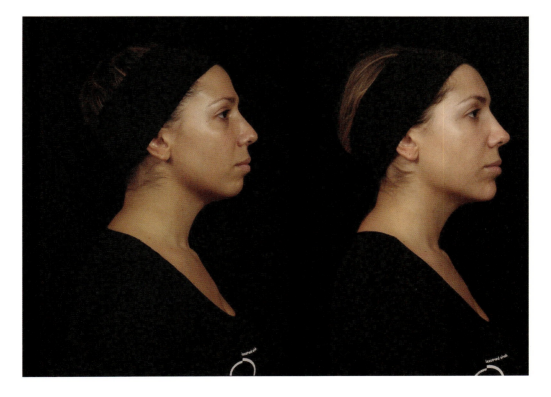

Patient 3 Figure 2 Side view of the female patient.

Patient 4: This was a male patient with nasal dorsum irregularities and associated microgenia. We injected 2 mL of very high G' filler on the nasal base (0.4 per side), anterior nasal spine (0.3 mL), nasal tip (0.1 mL), supratip area (0.15 mL), glabella (0.2 mL), and nasal dorsum (0.35 mL). We then performed a 2-mL

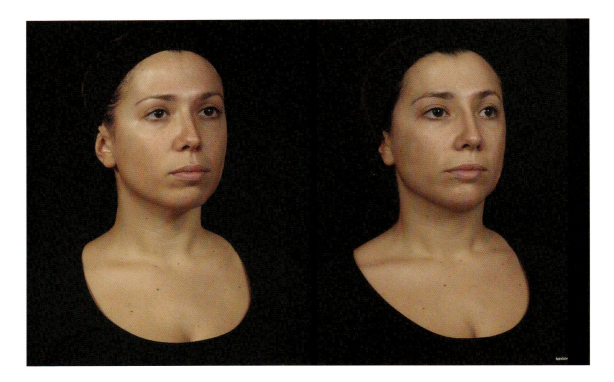

Patient 3 Figure 3 Three-quarters view of the female patient.

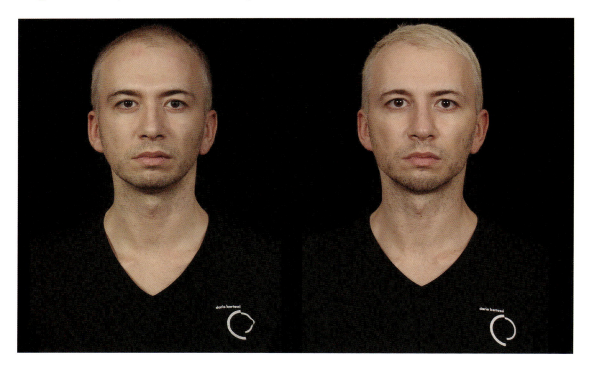

Patient 4 Figure 1 Front view of a male patient with asymmetric brow-tip aesthetic lines and microgenia: Improvement of the brow-tip aesthetic lines and chin projection.

injection on the midpoint of the chin, 1 mL on the lowest point of the chin bone, and 0.2 mL on the pogonion, as well as on the lateral points on the vertical line through the oral commissure on the bone along the jawline. We can appreciate the results before and after on the front (Figure 1), profile (Figure 2), and three-quarters view (Figure 3). The patient was satisfied with a good long-term result at 1 year postinjection.

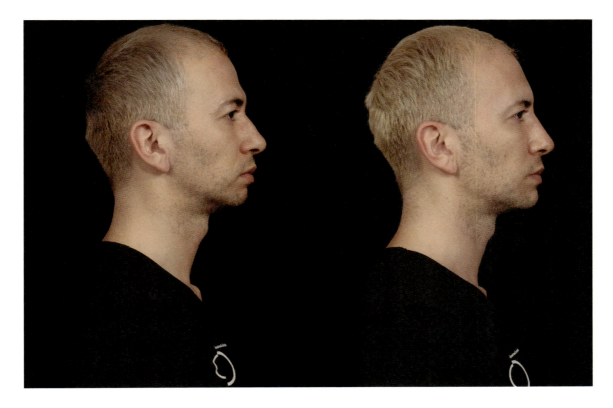

Patient 4 Figure 2 Side view of the male patient.

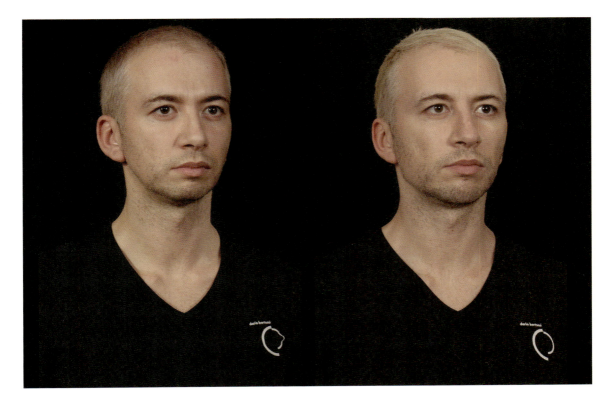

Patient 4 Figure 3 Three-quarters view of the male patient.

BIBLIOGRAPHY

1. Bertossi D, Malchiodi L, Albanese M, et al. Nonsurgical rhinoplasty with the novel hyaluronic acid filler VYC-25L: results using a nasal grid approach. Aesthet Surg J. 2021;41(6):NP512–NP520.
2. ASAPS: Cosmetic (aesthetic) surgery national data bank statistics, 2018. Available at: www.surgery.org/sites/default/files/ASAPS-Stats2018_0.pdf Accessed May 2022.
3. ASPS national clearinghouse of plastic surgery procedural statistics. Available at: www.plasticsurgery.org/documents/News/Statistics/2020/plastic-surgery-statistics-full-report-2020.pdf Accessed May 2022.
4. Kurkjian TJ, Ahmad J, Rohrich RJ. Soft-tissue fillers in rhinoplasty. Plast Reconstr Surg. 2014;133(2):121e–126e.
5. Kontis TC. The art of camouflage: when can a revision rhinoplasty be nonsurgical? Facial Plast Surg. 2018;34(3):270e277.
6. Hedén P. Nasal reshaping with hyaluronic acid: an alternative or complement to surgery. Plastic and Reconstructive Surgery—Global Open. 2016;4(11).
7. Callan P, Goodman GJ, Carlisle I, et al. Efficacy and safety of a hyaluronic acid filler in subjects treated for correction of midface volume deficiency: A 24 month study. Clin Cosmet Investig Dermatol. 2013;6:81–89.
8. Gold MH. Use of hyaluronic acid fillers for the treatment of the aging face. Clin Interv Aging. 2007;2(3):369–376.
9. Bray D, Hopkins C, Roberts DN. A review of dermal fillers in facial plastic surgery. Curr Opin Otolaryngol Head Neck Surg. 2010;18(4):295–302.
10. Goodman GJ, Bekhor P, Rich M, et al. A comparison of the efficacy, safety, and longevity of two different hyaluronic acid dermal fillers in the treatment of severe nasolabial folds: a multicenter, prospective, randomized, controlled, single-blind, within- subject study. Clin Cosmet Investig Dermatol. 2011;4:197–205.
11. Muhn C, Rosen N, Solish N, et al. The evolving role of hyaluronic acid fillers for facial volume restoration and contouring: a Canadian overview. Clin Cosmet Investig Dermatol. 2012;5:147–158.
12. Maloney BP. Nasal contouring using fillers. Operative Techniques in Otolaryngology. 2007;18:302–306.
13. Redaelli A. Medical rhinoplasty with hyaluronic acid and botulinum toxin A: a very simple and quite effective technique. J Cosmet Dermatol. 2008;7(3):210–220.
14. Xue K, Chiang CA, Liu K, et al. Multiplane hyal-uronic acid rhinoplasty. Plast Reconstr Surg. 2012;129(2):371e–372e.
15. Liew S, Scamp T, de Maio M, et al. Efficacy and safety of a hyaluronic acid filler to correct aesthetically detracting or deficient features of the Asian nose: A prospective, open-label, long-term study. Aesthet Surg J. 2016;36(7):760–772. Oxford University Press.
16. Rauso R, Colella G, Zerbinati N, Salti G. Safety and early satisfaction assessment of patients seeking nonsurgical rhinoplasty with filler. Journal of Cutaneous and Aesthetic Surgery. 2017;10(4):207–214.
17. Bertossi D, Lanaro L, Dell'Acqua I, et al. Injectable profiloplasty: forehead, nose, lips, and chin filler treatment. J Cosmet Dermatol. 2018;00:1–9.
18. Bertossi D, Lanaro L, Dorelan S, et al. Nonsurgical rhinoplasty: nasal grid analysis and nasal injecting protocol. Plastic and Reconstructive Surgery. 2019;143(2):428–439.
19. Youn SH, Seo KK. Filler rhinoplasty evaluated by anthropometric analysis. Dermatologic Surgery. 2016;42(9):1071–1081.
20. Tezel A, Fredrickson GH. The science of hyaluronic acid dermal fillers. J Cosmet Laser Ther. 2008;10(1):35–42.
21. Dayan SH, Bassichis BA. Facial dermal fillers: selection of appropriate products and techniques. Aesthet Surg J. 2008;28(3):335–347.
22. Carruthers J, Cohen SR, Joseph JH, et al. The science and art of dermal fillers for soft-tissue augmentation. J Drugs Dermatol. 2009;8:335–350.
23. Narins RS, Jewell M, Rubin M, et al. Clinical conference: management of rare events following dermal fillers—focal necrosis and angry red bumps. Dermatol Surg. 2006;32:426–434.
24. Rivkin A. A prospective study of non-surgical primary rhinoplasty using a polymethylmethacrylate injectable implant. Dermatol Surg. 2014;40:305–313.
25. Becker H. Nasal augmentation with calcium hydroxylapatite in a carrier-based gel. Plast Reconstr Surg. 2008;121:2142–2147.
26. Cassuto D. The use of Dermicol-P35 dermal filler for nonsurgical rhinoplasty. Aesthet Surg J. 2009;29(3 suppl):S22–S24.
27. Webster RC, Hamdan US, Gaunt JM, et al. Rhinoplastic revisions with injectable silicone. Arch Otolaryngol Head Neck Surg. 1986;112:269–276.
28. Siclovan HR, Jomah JA. Injectable calcium hydroxylapatite for correction of nasal bridge deformities. Aesthetic Plast Surg. 2009;33:544–548.
29. Jacovella PF, Peiretti CB, Cunille D, et al. Long-lasting results with hydroxyl-apatite (Radiesse) facial filler. Plast Reconstr Surg. 2006;118(3 suppl):15S–21S.
30. Jacovella PF. Aesthetic nasal corrections with hydroxylapatite facial filler. Plast Reconstr Surg. 2008;121:338e–339e.
31. Jacovella PF. Use of calcium hydroxylapatite (Radiesse) for facial augmentation. Clin Interv Aging. 2008;3(1):161–174.
32. Humphrey CD, Arkins JP, Dayan SH. Soft tissue fillers in the nose. Aesthet Surg J. 2009;29:477–484.
33. Rootman DB, Lin JL, Goldberg R. Does the Tyndall effect describe the blue hue periodically observed in subdermal hyaluronic acid gel placement? Ophthalmic Plast Reconstr Surg. 2014;30:524–527.
34. Singh P, Vijayan R, Nikkhah D. Filler rhinoplasty: Evidence, outcomes, and complications. Aesthet Surg J. 2018;38(11):NP165–NP167. Oxford University Press.

CHAPTER 7

Surrounding Areas

Ash Mohsaebi, Riccardo Nocini, and Ekaterina Gutop

INTRODUCTION

The anatomical profile and shape of the nose have a huge impact on the appearance and expressivity of the human face and are a major issue for facial symmetry; however, because the nose can be considered a complex anatomical three-dimensional shape, with critical roles and a critical impact for a harmonious and eye-catching appearance within the entire facial look, the areas surrounding the nose do not have a secondary or minor significance. The regions surrounding the nose account for a large number of fundamental issues characterizing the overall concept of the facial look; the overall intertwined ratios and dimensions between the nose and its surrounding regions affect the face's expressivity and its potential in social interactions. Skilled professionals frequently become expert at overall facial symmetry modeling within the human idea of beauty, as they need to address the aesthetic parameters of the human face as a whole from a surgical-anatomical perspective [1–4]. Non-surgical rhinoplasty should therefore not be limited to a narrowly defined nasal region, as surgeons and physicians can often enlist it in addition the numerous aesthetic techniques developed for the regions surrounding the nose.

It is noticeable that many facial anatomical variables and dimensional ratios concur altogether in shaping and/or altering the facial aesthetic look. Therefore, although rhinoplasty can be developed as an individualized practice, both a worldwide agreed upon standardization, founded on scientifically sound algorithms, and a consensus guideline should help operators to achieve a monitorable model of facial beauty, suggesting and organizing targeted plans to manage the most accurate logical progression of all those steps and leading to the development and stability of the overall available techniques. The ultimate target should always be an overall harmonious result involving the nose with its surrounding areas in order to result in a stunning or handsome face (Figure 7.1).

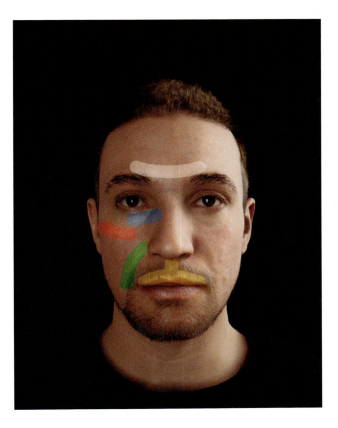

Figure 7.1 Overall harmonious result involving nose with surrounding areas.

NASAL SURROUNDING AREAS: CHEEK AND ZYGOMATIC ARCH

Both the cheek and the malar areas represent major aesthetic zones, which are usually the fundamental target of many cutting-edge aesthetic injectable approaches. The midface undergoes a deep evolution during aging. Current technology considers the aged midface the result of multifactorial causative factors, where bone structures, soft tissues, muscles, ligaments, adipose tissue and skin contribute together in various degrees to the typical aged look. A full comprehension of the principal matrix and tissue interactions is particularly important, as any compartment-associated change affects the interplay and the role of the major components in participating in an integral face rejuvenation [5–8].

From an anatomical point of view, the midface extends from the glabella to the subnasal region, where the malar area overlies the zygoma and malar bone. The nasal-labial area is exactly on the inferior edge and goes ahead on the horizontal line, which runs from the anterior nasal backbone to the insertion of the earlobe. The top boundary runs from the glabella to the higher margin of the zygomatic arch, following the infraorbital bone margin.

For treatment with HA fillers, the patient should be first evaluated in anterior, indirect, and lateral perspectives. The lateral evaluation is fundamental to assessing slight vectors within the midface. Furthermore, a deficient malar and midfacial projection usually emerges from the soft, poorly supporting tissues, resulting in a prematurely decreasing lip and cheek descent, eye bags, scleral display, and an evident aged look. These deficiencies should be assessed and insightfully addressed. Moreover, it is crucial to assess the facial look both at rest and in animation; upgrading in animation is typically predictive of a favorable outcome after correcting volumization [9,10]. The healthcare professional needs to carefully verify the function and synergy of the top-lip levators in order to enhance the intensity of placement, specifically when operating close to the chin.

For the zygoma at the lateral side, the only recommendation is to mark the lip-cheek junction (LCJ) with the patient in the upright "chin down, eyes up" position; this position accentuates the LCJ. The physician needs to palpate the zygomatic bone with two fingers and mark the superior and inferior borders meticulously. These are critical landmarks, as the middle temporal vein and transverse facial artery run parallel with the zygoma at 1 cm superiorly and inferiorly, respectively, to the bone. Faulty needle angulation involves the threat of vascular compromise. Then palpate and mark the suture between the zygomatic and frontal temporal bones. Again, mark two extra points 1 cm anteriorly and posteriorly to the suture if an additional lifting/guide is desired. Cleanse carefully, then retract the skin (while palpating the zygoma). Using a hollow needle for the injection is recommended in the interest of decreasing any concern about vascular complications. Aspirate for 4–6 seconds while stabilizing the needle tip; the time of the aspiration may vary, as it is dependent on the characteristics of the filler. Obviously, it is crucial to state that this approach cannot completely exclude the risk of an erroneously placed intravascular injection; both expert vigilance on the injection method and a slow injection pace and extrusion are mandatory. Then, inject a bolus anterior to the marking in the supraperiosteal plane, with the needle perpendicular to the bone. Be careful: Constantly be aware of the different moving regions, including the glabella and the nasal tip. If a medical assessment confirms it is suitable, the physician should set a hyaluronic acid (HA) bolus additionally in the anterior and then the posterior part of the first point. Palpate and mark the malar eminence, then inject a supraperiosteal bolus, applying the injection technique as for the lateral malar point.

Finally, for the midcheek, the area can be volumized according to three straightforward ranges, depending on the clinical targets, namely at the bone, inside the deep medial cheek fat pads (DMCF), and inside the medial suborbicularis oculi fat (SOOF). A proper medical assessment of suitability is of utmost importance, as product placement above the top-lip levators may also elongate the top lip; their movement is probably enhanced in terms of efficiency if the filler is put underneath the levators. A greater lifting impact may be achieved through injection to the lateral part of the cheek bone, below the zygomatic ligament. Using a cannula for the lateral part of the zygomatic arch is recommended in order to limit any possible harm to the superficial temporal artery. Once the cannula has been correctly inserted from the targeted part of the cheek, it should commence with each lateral side, then with the medial part of the zygomatic proximity, and then the procedure can be performed around the specific layers. Moreover, the surgeon can proceed to perform a certain amount of traction of the soft tissues, both laterally and superiorly, on the basis of proper knowledge of the layer of insertion and careful and cautious injection on the supraperiosteal or the DMCF plane with a cannula; this should result in improvement and lifting when the outcome is not optimal in the corrected site itself, and this result can also be achieved in the areas surrounding it. Performing the injection in a dynamic modality—for instance, upon smiling—can help prevent any overcorrection.

Even a defect of the anteromedial part of the midface and midcheek groove may be a target for correction. In this case, the zygomatic area should be treated from the lateral to the medial side, with a needle, a cannula, or both. By treating the lateral part first, an improvement in the anteromedial part of the midface can be achieved. From the insertion point, positioned beneath the projection of the malar eminence, the HA product may be injected at the deep supraperiosteal or DMCF pad plane. Correction of the midcheek groove alone may be an indication for correcting with an overfilling or "sausage" effect in this region. A cannula is preferred because of the position of the infraorbital foramen.

The surrounding nasal area consists of the infraorbital sector, which has an important impact on appearance. The perception of tiredness in this anatomical region has to be addressed at the cheek and zygomatic arch by correcting the deficiency in bone structures and fat pads with filler. A direct approach for the infraorbital location is highly encouraged, and using a cannula helps to reduce the danger of vascular-related headaches.

A pleasing aesthetic outcome is completed via the use of a cannula from the insertion point, placed at the projection of the malar eminence, sliding along the lower orbital rim by using the cannula, and injecting filler with lower hydrophilic features beneath the orbicularis retaining ligament (ORL). An ideal result to avoid overcorrection can be achieved by the "micro bolus" technique, with a limited amount of filler (less than 0.3 mL) for the medial element and 0.5 mL for the lateral, with the effect of an undercorrection. If there is to be a complete, thorough correction immediately after, that can be a reason for overfilling inside the periorbital sector.

In the case of botulinum toxin, avoid putting toxins for the lateral canthus inferior to the superior zygomatic arch, as these can spread into the zygomaticus major and minor muscle groups, with subsequent ipsilateral facial paralysis or lip ptosis. Overtreatment of the lateral canthus decreases the function of the orbicularis oculi as the best elevator of the cheek and might increase the risk of palpebral edema in predisposed people. To avoid inadvertent treatment of risorius, with a consequent uneven smile, remain in the safe region of 1 cm from the anterior border of masseter when treating the masseter with botulinum toxin [11–13].

NASAL SURROUNDING AREAS: NASOLABIAL REGION

Although the terms "wrinkle" and "fold" are frequently used interchangeably, they describe different entities [14,15]. The nasolabial wrinkle or crease is a sharp, linear fold defining the border between the top lip and the cheek. The nasolabial fold (NLF) is observed laterally to the wrinkle as a bulge which extends from the nasal ala to the eyelash proximity.

Although the intensity and density of the nasolabial wrinkle may vary depending on race, sex, age, and weight, the wrinkle itself usually starts developing slightly laterally to the ala of the nose and should end 1–2 cm laterally to the mouth angle. Although it is sometimes thought that the nasolabial wrinkle is a pure cutaneous fold, it has been documented to be a true anatomical border between the cheek, which has a beneficial layer of subcutaneous fat, and the lip, in which both pores and skin are firmly attached to the orbicularis muscle with no interposed fascia [16,17]. The nasolabial wrinkle can therefore be defined as the sharp line demarcating the start of the greater laterally placed NLF. The softening of the wrinkle optically reduces the severity of the NLF, but a deeper nasolabial wrinkle, observed by way of an extra bulging fold, contributes to a more aged look.

The nasolabial wrinkle is likewise of utmost importance in facial features. There are conflicting theories as to the formation of this nasolabial wrinkle—a muscular and a fascial concept. The muscular theory maintains that the nasolabial wrinkle is formed predominantly by the muscle-dermal insertions of the top lip levators. The fascial theory maintains that the nasolabial wrinkle is fashioned largely due to dense fibrous tissue and the firm fascial attachments into the fascia of the lip elevator muscle tissues. Beer et al. [18] reported evidence for the muscular theory. They dissected and harvested the nasolabial wrinkles from 14 hemi-facial dissections and showed numerous skeletal muscle fibers in the epidermis. In addition, dermal muscle fibers were reported at 4 mm medial and 4 mm lateral to the nasolabial wrinkle, yet in amounts considerably less than directly inside the wrinkle. They finally demonstrated that the use of low doses of intradermal botulinum toxin located directly inside the nasolabial wrinkle may help to decrease or maybe eradicate the wrinkle itself, and thereby the NLF, because of the residual local muscle fibers across the wrinkle itself.

Sandulescu et al. recently assessed the fascial theory. After a careful dissection, sophisticated three-dimensional reconstructions of the histological structures were carried out, together with scanning electron microscope (SEM) analysis of the NLF [14–16]. They observed that there may be an NLF superficial musculoaponeurotic system (SMAS)—a fibromuscular, three-dimensional meshwork bolstered with fat cells. An unexpected porosity and an SMAS-like system were identified as close or adjoining to the NLF. The SMAS structure in the cheek confirmed a quite normal, vertically parallel alignment of fibrous septa, which generates a type of three-dimensional meshwork of interrelated compartments. The morphology is altered by being condensed while in transit over the NLF to form an abnormal structure in the upper lip location. SEM showed the association between the fibrous meshwork and the adipose cells. Blood microflows inside the SMAS circulation extended underneath, inside the subcutaneous tissue, without causing perforation into the fibromuscular septa.

There is also a further osseous aspect involving the NLF. Several years after his first presentation, Pessa studied computed tomography (CT) scans of patients with persistent pain and discovered that skeletal maxillary/orbital top adjustments indicated a deeper NLF [19, 20].

Finally, the skin also plays a function in the appearance of the NLF. In the older affected patient, the number of pores and the excess skin above the fold accentuate an aged look. This appearance can derive both from an actual skin excess or from a pseudo-excess due to facial fat atrophy, specifically in the midface location. In particular, the NLF divides an area with a correct amount of subcutaneous fat (cheek) and an area with minimum fat. The fold derives from a number of factors, which include muscular activity, SMAS, fat, bone, and skin; for this reason, there may be no single approach to correct the NLF.

When intending to use a hyaluronic acid (HA) filler, the medical professional should conduct a careful whole-face assessment and then proceed to fix underlying bone and smooth tissue elements contributing to sagging, always first addressing the causative elements and the lateral facial vectors before moving on to improve the nasolabial area itself. An indirect method may consist of the treatment of the zygomatic arch, bone, and submalar area according to the symptoms and with the perfect amount and proper features of the filler. Then the medical professional must assess the higher, mid-, and lower third of the NLF while planning treatment. Inside the nasolabial area, the facial artery is retrievable within the middle layer of tissue and needs to be specifically recognized and kept clear of being touched. Consequently, injections are accomplished inside the superficial reticular epidermis or more deeply, reaching the bone floor. Within the superior part of the NLF, the motion is deep (as far as the pyriform fossa), via a needle. Cleanse with particular attention and maintain strict aseptic technique. Then aim down from the nasal ala towards the alternative oral commissure, stopping at the pyriform bone, and aspirate; do not inject if the tip is not on the bone. By contrast, the top NLF is superficial (reached with either a needle or a cannula); you should be aware that placement has to be in the reticular dermis or immediate subcutis.

Botulinum toxin injected intradermally within the NLF reduces its depth, probably due to the fact that medial and lateral dermal muscle fibers are close to each other. Kane [21] described the use of botulinum toxin injected into muscle tissue related to the dynamic conduct of the NLF. In certain patients, mimetic muscular tissues around the NLF have cutaneous insertions in the fold, making it an unusual procedure in patients from their teens to 35 years of age. A gummy smile may also be ameliorated. However, in the case of ptosis of the soft tissues, botulinum toxin in the mimetic muscles is of limited use.

NASAL SURROUNDING AREAS: LIPS

Lips and their anatomical place are aesthetic fundamental components of the facial look and therefore play a paramount role within facial rejuvenation methods; lips and eyes have historically been highlighted as the two most beautiful regions of the human face [22]. Not only are the lips an important part of the primary facial triangle, they also play a crucial position in sensual enchantment, facial expression, articulation, and masticatory competence. Lips also help oral sealing and define the limits of the teeth by means of soft tissues. Each lip has its appropriate form; the composition and the thickness of each lower and upper lip may also fluctuate appreciably, simply because differences include many genetic components, even inside one ethnicity. In Caucasian patients, the top lip normally appears narrower than the bottom, in a ratio expected to be 40:60. In African and Afro-American patients the ratio is 50:50 [23]. The enhancement of lips by way of cosmetic procedures entails reshaping and amplifying the top and bottom lips in order to enhance the three-dimensional relationship with the nose, teeth, and surrounding facial systems at rest, in addition to adjusting the lips for the duration of any facial motion and speech.

A deep understanding of lip anatomy, bearing in mind their perioral location, is crucial for excellent and safe lip rejuvenation. The so-called Cupid's bow incorporates two paramedial elevations along the top vermilion border. The philtrum incorporates two raised vertical philtrum columns adjoining to a midline separation. In the elderly, photodamage, hereditary factors, and smoking contribute to volume loss, perioral rhytids, and the prominence of labiomental folds. There are numerous indications for the remedy of the perioral region as part of the surrounding nasal areas; however, the final result of the correction should be harmonious with the rest of the face in all perspectives. To maintain harmony, the lips must be handled as the final step within the complete plan of facial adjustments. Deficiency of quantity for the young patient is certainly one of the important indications for lip correction.

Skinny lips deriving from genetic causes or an asymmetric face may be addressed by augmenting smooth tissues around the lips. Features of the youthful lip consist of clean pores and skin without visible rhytids straight away above the vermillion border, sharply described philtral columns, a well-described Cupid's bow, a top lip with an outstanding medial tubercle with bilateral depressions, a bottom lip with a corresponding small fold centrally, and lateral protrusions. On the lateral profile, the top cutaneous "white" lip should be brief with a concavity near the vermillion lip. The top lip needs to venture only slightly outside the bottom (about 2 mm). Attractive female lips tend to have an improved vermillion top, an elevated nasolabial perspective, and an improved labiomental angle [24–28]. In elderly patients pores and skin look older and there usually is thinning of the bottom and top lips, an elongated shape of the top lip, and wrinkles inside the perioral area.

For the use of botulinum toxin, ensure the patient has practical expectations: the toxin will tone down dynamic perioral wrinkles but will not eradicate wrinkles seen at rest. An extra amelioration can be achieved by the use of a mixture of fillers and energy-based devices. Start with incremental doses in order not to influence phonation and articulation, especially in singers and public speakers. Bear in mind doubling the dilution of toxin to enhance its ability to be distributed. A cumulative 4–6 U dosage from a variety of onabotulinum toxin is generally recommended for lip treatment, inside each top and each bottom lip. Ice, topical anesthesia, or vibration may relieve the pain upon injection.

For the use of the HA filler, there are some strategies to be highlighted. In the linear threading technique, the health practitioner typically accomplishes the approach in a retrograde way, with filler being injected on withdrawal of the needle or cannula. Anterograde technique refers to filler being extruded even as the needle is advanced; this method can be safer than other strategies because the filler, flowing forwards to the needle tip, pushes vessels out of the way, thus minimizing tissue trauma and the possibility of an intravascular injection.

The primary injection sites for fillers are:

1. The vermilion border, where a retrograde threading technique is used. The cutaneous pores and skin should not be injected to avoid a sharp and overdefined lip contour, which can also bring about unnatural fullness of the vermilion border and further elongation of the cutaneous top lip.
2. The perioral rhytids, where a retrograde threading is used with a 30G needle positioned immediately within the line. With this approach, it is possible to correct static and dynamic lines.
3. The philtral columns. Insert the needle on the top of the two humps with the aid of the Cupid's bow, in the direction of the nasal septum. Then consider using a slow retrograde threading approach and pinch the skin with the non-dominant hand during the injection to save lateral splaying. At the end of the retrograde injection, a small amount of gel can also be deposited to provide a boost to the Cupid's bow and aid the projection of the crucial top lip.

In the fan-shaped approach, the technique is likewise linear threading, involving longitudinal insertion of the needle and extruding the HA filler upon withdrawal of the needle. However, the needle should now not be completely removed, but diverted to a new filling point. The filler is thus injected along several short lines with the advantage of fewer access points and less tissue trauma.

The most frequent injection site is the vermilion body. In this case, it is essential to start injection from this region, which minimizes the risk of excessive correction and improves the appearance of the associated perioral radial rhytides. Injection should be performed starting from the mucosal side of the lip by inserting at 45 degrees or otherwise using a cannula to reduce the possibility of bruising and swelling from different points. The injection must then be directed towards the center with a 20-degree perspective, changing direction each time to offer a homogeneous and complete filling.

With the serial puncture approach, the method involves a couple of close injections. It is very helpful to pull the skin slightly away and out to keep the skin taut during injections. Multiple carefully spaced gel deposits need to be located, and in the case of postinjection gaps, regular rubbing is required to mix the filler. This approach allows for a unique squeeze and placement of the extra fill. The characteristics of the filler should be carefully considered: the aim is an HA product with low and medium cohesion characteristics. However, there remains a possibility of accelerated bruising and swelling due to accelerated tissue trauma. The main injection site for this approach is the vermilion border, treated by injecting at a 30-degree angle with the peak of the cutaneous upper lip to beautify the site itself and correct some short perioral rhytides.

CONCLUSIONS

We should consider the nasal structure essential to achieve an excellent aesthetic appearance with the fulfilment of a harmonious face, and this calls for an evaluation of all areas close to the nose as well. Assessing the ideal anatomy of the facial site as a whole and comparing the dynamic interaction between anatomy and features is of paramount importance.

To achieve a very high aesthetic result, different strategies may need to be used, surgical or non-surgical remedies. Non-surgical strategies can offer reduced morbidity compared to surgery and improve skin pleasantness and texture with minimal danger to the patient. These non-surgical techniques are powerful and have a quick recovery time for properly managed patients, allowing them to resume their lifestyles again very rapidly. However, despite these indisputable advantages, non-surgical whole facial treatments are often not recommended or are recommended only due to their more accessible nature. The approach using non-surgical treatments is divided into more than one clinical session, and there needs to be a correct assessment of the facial areas, combined with a high level of scientific experience, to obtain the best result.

Many pharmaceutical modalities achieve a stunning face as a result; however, the strategies to quantify and standardize the drugs are still burdensome. Consequently, the relationships between unique anatomical regions, internally mounted parameters or canonical ranges, and volumes and shapes should be considered in detail to achieve the precise intended purpose. The technique of separating the face into small portions with a grid allows the physician to recognize the constrained regions to be treated. It greatly improves the ability to correct defects and restore an appropriate proportion of different anatomical components of the front and profile views, with the aim of making the treated patient beautiful.

BIBLIOGRAPHY

1. Guyuron B. Dynamic interplays during rhinoplasty. Clin Plast Surg. 1996 Apr;23(2):223–231.
2. Lam SM, Williams EF 3rd. Anatomic considerations in aesthetic rhinoplasty. Facial Plast Surg. 2002 Nov;18(4):209–214.
3. Sykes JM. Management of the middle nasal third in revision rhinoplasty. Facial Plast Surg. 2008 Aug;24(3):339–347.
4. Totonchi A, Guyuron B. The external rhinoplasty approach. Clin Plast Surg. 2022 Jan;49(1):49–59.
5. Rohrich RJ, Avashia YJ, Savetsky IL. Prediction of facial aging using the facial fat compartments. Plast Reconstr Surg. 2021 Jan 1;147(1S-2):38S–42S.
6. Mendelson B, Wong CH. Changes in the facial skeleton with aging: implications and clinical applications in facial rejuvenation. Aesthetic Plast Surg. 2020 Aug;44(4):1151–1158.
7. Mendelson BC, Wong CH. Changes in the facial skeleton with aging: implications and clinical applications in facial rejuvenation. Aesthetic Plast Surg. 2020 Aug;44(4):1159–1161.
8. Shaw RB Jr, Katzel EB, Koltz PF, et al. Facial bone density: effects of aging and impact on facial rejuvenation. Aesthet Surg J. 2012 Nov;32(8):937–942.
9. Pozner JN. Novel injection technique for Malar Cheek volume restoration. Aesthetic Plast Surg. 2018 Oct;42(5):1393.
10. Shamban A, Clague MD, von Grote E, Nogueira A. A novel and more aesthetic injection pattern for Malar Cheek volume restoration. Aesthetic Plast Surg. 2018 Feb;42(1):197–200.
11. Zhou R, Fei Y, Sun L, et al. BTX-a rejuvenation: regional botulinum toxin-A injection of the platysma in patients with facial sagging. Aesthetic Plast Surg. 2019 Aug;43(4):1044–1053.
12. Patel PN, Owen SR, Norton CP, et al. Outcomes of buccinator treatment with botulinum toxin in facial synkinesis. JAMA Facial Plast Surg. 2018 May 1;20(3):196–201.
13. Sapra P, Demay S, Sapra S, et al. A single-blind, split-face, randomized, pilot study comparing the effects of intradermal and intramuscular injection of two commercially available botulinum toxin a formulas to reduce signs of facial aging. J Clin Aesthet Dermatol. 2017 Feb;10(2):34–44.
14. Sandulescu T, Franzmann M, Jast J, et al. Facial fold and crease development: a new morphological approach and classification. Clin Anat. 2019 May;32(4):573–584.
15. Sandulescu T, Stoltenberg F, Buechner H, et al. Platysma and the cervical superficial musculoaponeurotic system—comparative analysis of facial crease and platysmal band development. Ann Anat. 2020 Jan;227:151414.
16. Sandulescu T, Buechner H, Rauscher D, et al. Histological, SEM and three-dimensional analysis of the midfacial SMAS—new morphological insights. Ann Anat. 2019 Mar;222:70–78.
17. Velazco de Maldonado GJ, Suárez-Vega DV, et al. Innovative paradigm in aesthetics medicine: proposal for diagnostic morphological geometric by thirds, semiology in clinical applied to aging facial. J Cutan Aesthet Surg. 2020 Apr–Jun;13(2):112–123.
18. Beer KR. Handbook of botulinum toxin for aesthetic indications. In Theory and practice. London: JP Medical Pract; 2016, pp. 1–123.
19. Pessa JE, Nguyen H, John GB, Scherer PE. Aesthet Surg J. 2014 Feb;34(2):227–34. doi: 10.1177/1090820X13517896. Epub 2013 Dec 18. PMID: 24353247.
20. Farkas JP, Pessa JE, Hubbard B, Rohrich RJ. The science and theory behind facial aging. Plast Reconstr Surg Glob Open. 2013 May 7;1(1):e8–e15.
21. Kane MA. The effect of botulinum toxin injections on the nasolabial fold. Plast Reconstr Surg. 2003 Oct;112(5 Suppl):66S–72S; discussion 73S–74S.
22. Trevidic P. Ageing of the lips. In Azib N, Charrier JB, Cornette de Saint-Cyr B et al., eds. Anatomy and lip enhancement. E2e Medical; 2013, p. 9.
23. Alexis AF, Few J, Callender VD, et al. Myths and knowledge gaps in the aesthetic treatment of patients with skin of color. J Drugs Dermatol. 2019 Jul 1;18(7):616–622.
24. Frâncu LL, Hînganu D, Hînganu MV. Anatomical evidence regarding the existence of sustentaculum facies. Rom J Morphol Embryol. 2013;54(3 Suppl):757–761.
25. Kaminer MS, Cohen JL, Shamban A, et al. Maximizing panfacial aesthetic outcomes: findings and recommendations from the HARMONY study. Dermatol Surg. 2020 Jun;46(6):810–817. doi: 10.1097/DSS.0000000000002271.
26. Surek CC. Facial anatomy for filler injection: the Superficial Musculoaponeurotic System (SMAS) is not just for facelifting. Clin Plast Surg. 2019 Oct;46(4):603–612. doi: 10.1016/j.cps.2019.06.007.
27. Kapoor KM, Murthy R, Hart SLA, et al. Factors influencing pre-injection aspiration for hyaluronic acid fillers: a systematic literature review and meta-analysis. Dermatol Ther. 2021 Jan;34(1):e14360. doi: 10.1111/dth.14360.
28. Carruthers A, Carruthers J, Hardas B, et al. A validated facial grading scale: the future of facial ageing measurement tools? J Cosmet Laser Ther. 2010;12(5):235–241.

CHAPTER **8**

Non-Surgical Profileplasty

Thierry Besins, Ali Pirayesh, and Dario Bertossi

INTRODUCTION

There have been remarkable achievements in the developmental pathways leading to improvement in aesthetic medicine: one such development has been the perspective of addressing the whole facial plane (the so-called "full-face approach"), where it is of utmost importance to consider the best anatomical-functional relationship among different parts—the nose, forehead, chin, and submental region [1–3]. Although many researchers have adopted defined parameters in their approach to the profile, which should lead to "a beautiful" profile line, the results may not always be as expected [1–7], as the treatment of a single facial area in isolation rather than a whole-face treatment can lead to less-than-satisfactory results [3]. (Moreover, judging the facial profile is not a constant entity, as factors such as age, ethnicity, and culture may thoroughly revise the way it is interpreted.)

Another development is that non-surgical aesthetic treatment of the human face is now considered an affordable alternative to surgical invasive procedures, allowing the physician to save time, reduce expenditure burdens, and prevent hazards and complications. The treatment planning of facial aesthetic changes is currently challenging, and the literature to date provides only a fragmented description of profile treatment with hyaluronic acid (HA) fillers [8–10]. Most of them focus separately on each limited area [11–16], rather than on the simultaneous treatment of the forehead, nose, lips, chin, and submental area. However, medical profileplasty allows the physician to attain relevant aesthetic results after just a single session; the simultaneous correction to the forehead, nose, lips, chin, and submental area leads to an overall improvement in facial aesthetics and harmony, avoiding scars and costs deriving from general anesthesia. This methodology is set to become a leading practice in achieving the global, coordinated, and time-efficient achievement of a beautiful facial appearance.

INJECTABLE PROFILEPLASTY

To achieve consistently good results, the best recommendation is to implement the following practices:

1. Accurate case selection, which implies recognizing the coexistence of defects in the nose and chin.
2. An accurate pretreatment evaluation with pictures, which analyzes how and how much to revise and correct.
3. Scheduling a correct sequence treatment, such as forehead, nose, lips, and chin (moreover, a useful top-down sequence that provides a good profile setting).

A comprehensive clinical facial trait analysis should be used to enhance the diagnosis, treatment planning, and quality of results (see Figure 8.1). The Arnett analysis in soft tissues could provide a tool to optimally investigate and fix aesthetic disharmonies. If the analysis of soft tissues following Arnett's parameters is thoroughly adopted in non-surgical profileplasty, the surgeon may be able to assess many fundamental steps to better perform a clinical evaluation [3, 17]. Taking as the reference the true vertical line (TVL), a line running from the subnasal point in the natural head position (NHP) [17,18], the surgeon usually monitors the sagittal pre- and posttreatment distance of the following soft tissue points: forehead (F), glabella (Gb), nasion (Na), nasal dorsum (Nd), nasal tip (Nt), subnasal (Sn), upper lip anterior (ULA), lower lip anterior (LLA), soft tissue point B (B), pogonion (Pg), and gnathion (Gn) [3].

Ricketts described the ideal position of the lower lip to 2 mm behind the E-line [19], whereas Merrifield described an angle between the Frankfurt plane and profile line formed by touching the chin and the foremost lip [20]. Some years later, Scheideman studied the anteroposterior point on the soft tissues and the vertical relationships of facial soft tissues [21]. Moreover, Burstone

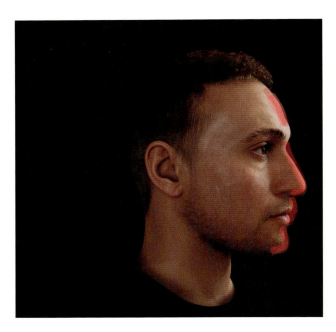

Figure 8.1 Profile areas to be treated according to the nasal defect.

studied lip assessment to create a correct proportion between the interlabial gap and the lower face height [22]. It appears that to date an accurate method of facial profiling has not yet been devised. For these reasons, some authors proposed the soft tissue Arnett facial analysis for diagnosis and treatment planning, using a simple and systematic method to both HA injection in the forehead, nose, lips, and chin and deoxycholic acid (DA) injections in the submental area with the purpose of correcting profile defects [3].

Picture analysis allows us to identify many defects, among which are the:

1. Overall facial profile view proportions
2. Forehead shape
3. Type of nose deformity, i.e., nasal hump, defective nasal projection, acute nasolabial angle, hidden columella or tip drooping, crooked nose, deep radix of the nose, saddle nose, nasal base asymmetry
4. Type of chin deformity, such as sagittal defect, vertical defect, and mixed defect

One possible technique is to select a product made by HA cross-linked with Vycross technology and DA, without anesthesia. After skin disinfection with 75% alcoholic solution, injection is performed with a top-down method, from the top (forehead) to the bottom (submental area). Treatment is usually performed using coded injection points to minimize vascular risks and complications.

Nowadays, the non-surgical approach offers different choices to our patients. Non-surgical profileplasty allows the physician to avoid general anesthesia, splints, swelling, and bruising and allows patients to return to work in a very short period (e.g., the same or the next day). The filler should be resorbable to avoid undesired complications such as granuloma, nodules, dislocation, allergies, and long-term palpability [3]. Furthermore, non-surgical techniques allow the physician to avoid typical surgical complications such as wide muscular detachment, osteotomy, and the risk of permanent paresthesia.

Forehead surgical treatment may involve also nano-fat injection, osteoplasty, or prosthesis insertion in the temporal or frontal region. Compared to filler treatment, all those procedures are affected by an increased incidence of edema and superinfections. However, osteoplasty or any procedure of prosthesis insertion (with its expected incision and scar) is increasingly less accepted by patients. Rhino-filler is also an increasingly used alternative for the set of patients who are reluctant to have permanent surgery; for them, fillers provide a non-permanent dissolvable trial. They also offer a solution to correct asymmetry and imperfections in 5–15% of affected postoperative rhinoplasty patients. Reports can be retrieved from the major professional societies (American Society for Aesthetic Plastic Surgery [ASAPS] [23] and American Society of Plastic Surgeons [ASPS]) that show a decrease in the popularity of surgical rhinoplasty and a concurrent increase in the use of fillers.

As the procedure becomes more generally requested, it is crucial and paramount to develop a reproducible, logically sequenced, safety-based protocol for both training and injecting purposes. Moreover, mental filler associated with submental DA injections, compared to chin osteotomy and submental liposuction, usually demonstrates a reduction in complications from mild paresthesia in at least 30% of the surgical patients at day 1 post-op to no sensory defects [3, 23–26].

SURGICAL PROFILEPLASTY

As detailed earlier, the assessment of the whole face for the relationship between the forehead, nose, lips, chin, and submental space, in the context of an evaluation of facial aesthetics, is becoming more and more popular and should be considered the key to successful aesthetic outcomes. As previously assessed, profile judgment cannot be considered an undisputable entity. It will change the appearance; however, a variety of ages, ethnicities, cultural beliefs, and fashion trends are involved, and although many researchers have sought parameters to follow that would lead to "a beautiful" profile line, the results may not always be as anticipated.

A weak chin, inadequate lower facial height, or submental fullness can lead to less-than-satisfactory results when performing any isolated correction with long intervals. An accurate facial analysis may report a significant number of patients requesting primary or secondary profile improvement, who even present with upper, mid, and lower face defects. There is a huge number of surgical techniques to achieve a complete profileplasty, such as surgical forehead correction, rhinoplasty, lip lipofilling, genioplasty, and submental liposuction. Forehead correction is a standard aesthetic surgical operation, wherein all the forehead skin region may be stretched, or we may insert grafts or inject fat. Rhinoplasty is one of the most used techniques, either in association with other procedures or alone. It is possible to assess the same issue for lip correction through lipofilling and for genioplasty, which is an ancillary procedure found to be useful in many circumstances. Submental liposuction is now a frequent procedure in aesthetic facial surgery.

The methodological approach for the forehead includes a surgical lift. In this case, a preoperative design is done with the patient in a sitting position. The incision line is designed individually depending on the patient enrolled. The surgery is performed under general anesthesia, with subsequent injection of 2% lidocaine with 1:100,000 epinephrine 100–150 mL of tumescent solution along the planned incision line and the periorbital area. The dissection is performed cutting just through the supraperiosteal layer to the superior orbital rim, paying careful attention to avoid injury to the deep branch of the supraorbital nerve. The ligaments in the periorbital region should be detached sufficiently to achieve the elevation of the eyebrow. Then the supraorbital neurovascular bundle, supratrochlear nerve, corrugator muscle, depressor supracilii muscle, and nasal root are exposed carefully, and the corrugator and procerus muscles are removed partially. In the case of crow's feet, an incision of the orbicularis oculi muscle is performed using an electric knife. To allow better adhesion of the elevated flap to the bed, areolar tissue and parts of the frontal periosteum are removed and the excess flap is excised. Scalp incisions are closed into one layer using skin staplers. When closing the hairline incision, subcutaneous and skin sutures are performed with 5-0 and 3-0 Vicryl and 6-0 nylon, respectively.

Application of the procedure may vary in light of different and particular features of the individual patients; additionally, the use of fat grafting can be included in the process. After harvesting 10 mL of fat, injection is performed with a 1-mL Luer-Lok syringe and 3-mm Byron cannula in the deep temporal fossa over the periosteum and the subgaleal plane with the fat tissue distributing an average of 2–3 mL per side in the temple and the remaining 4 mL on the central forehead.

For the nose, exclusion criteria are previous rhinoplasties, normal skin thickness and texture, previous trauma, scars, functional problems, and metabolic and hematological problems. All nose corrections are made using an open approach. Patients are usually treated with a cephalic resection of the lateral crura, generally leaving at least 8 mm as a residual strip. The nasal tips are treated with an intradomal suture with PDS 5-0 to remodel the tip. In all patients we perform medial oblique osteotomies and lateral curved basal osteotomies. Steri-Strips with Mastisol for 7 days with thermoplastic packing may be applied, and then Steri-Strips only for a further 7 days. At 2 and 12 months after surgery, scar healing is evaluated. Sometimes, residual inferior alveolar nerve (IAN) paresthesia is observed with a second neurosensorial test, and in this case the bone remodeling is checked by means of panoramic x-ray and tele-radiography in lateral and in frontal projection. Postoperative photos are usually included. By comparing pre- and postoperative photos, we have a complete overview of the healing process, and by comparing x-rays, we can record the exact changes in the patient's facial structures.

For lips, lipofilling is used and three injections of autologous fat are included. The lip points are identified as upper and lower vermilion, philtrum columns, upper and lower lip body, and right and left oral commissure. Without performing local anesthesia and using a 21G cannula of 5 cm length (TSK Laboratory Europe B.V. The Netherlands), 0.4 mL per side of autologous fat can be injected.

In the case of the chin, all procedures are performed under general anesthesia. Usually, the oral vestibule is injected with 2% xylocaine 1:100,000 mixed with a 1:1 ratio of physiologic solution, waiting 15 minutes for vasoconstriction. An incision line is made between the two canines using the 15-blade scalpel 6 mm below the attached mucosa; the surgeon then proceeds with the electric scalpel to the bone surface. Soft tissue detachment is performed. Then, the surgeon proceeds by exposing the periosteum and doing bone markings with a pencil and then holes with a drill. Marking the midline is particularly useful when, after the osteotomy, while performing the advancement you have to fix the osteotomized segment in a symmetrical position. Skin marks are made in order to have an immediate comparison with bone marks. Osteotomies and ostectomies are performed with a reciprocating saw. Bone segment fixation is done by means of titanium mini-plates and screws. Following fixation, before mucosal closure, mentalis muscle reattachment is carried out to avoid chin pad and cervical layer ptosis. A 4-0 Vicryl suture for muscle and 5-0 Vicryl suture for the mucosa is used. Elastic tissue adhesive band is applied to the chin for 2 days to reduce edema and to prevent hematoma formation by preventing soft tissue ptosis and residual asymmetries. The day after surgery a clinical neurosensorial test is performed to evaluate IAN function.

The submental liposuction is then carried out through a small 3-mm incision under the jaw. Usually, 5 mL of saline solution and Naropin (L-bupivacaine) (1:1) is infiltrated. The excess preplatysma fat is aspirated through 4-mm liposuction cannulas, and improvement of the contour of chin and neckline is accomplished. Postoperative complications like bruising, swelling, contour irregularities, dimpling, para- or hypoesthesia, and temporary motor nerve weakness are surgeon-dependent. The whole procedure usually takes about 15 minutes, and patients are asked to wear a chin strap for 7 days after the procedure. The recovery lasts 7–10 days, and patients can generally return to work within 1 week, but patients must be aware that the real result is gained after 3–4 months.

A forehead lift is a procedure that allows one to achieve a huge movement of the forehead's soft tissues. It is true that it is an expensive and invasive procedure that is loaded with serious complications; on the other hand, it is useful when you have to achieve a big movement.

Fat grafting of the forehead is a technique that has been used for 100 years. It is a mini-invasive procedure, and it allows a stable result if compared with HA fillers. About 30% of every single fat injection remains in the injection site, depending on the quality of the layer. This fact, in association with the lower grade of complications, makes this technique the first choice in forehead treatment.

In recent years the increase in requests for rhinoplasty has brought new procedures such as the use of an HA filler. This can be a good choice of treatment, but it is loaded with severe complications like necrosis of the nasal tip or, in the worst case, loss of vision. Conventional open rhinoplasty is a procedure that allows the range of nasal modification; you can modify soft tissues. This allows great results, in particular in posttraumatic rhinoplasty; moreover, open rhinoplasty increases respiratory performance when it is needed.

Lip surgery with the fat grafting technique is one of the oldest procedures in aesthetic surgery. Like the lipofilling of the forehead region, it allows stable results and non-invasive treatment.

Furthermore, to date, chinplasty is an easy surgical procedure, and it can be performed by means of an osteotomy or by positioning alloplastic materials, but some controversies have yet to be addressed. We prefer the intraoral approach with an incision line running between the two canines and believe that the intraoral approach should be the only one considered for osteotomies. Zide and McCarthy postulated the importance of the mentalis muscle in chin surgery [27], and Chaushu showed that when mentalis muscle insertion is not precisely repositioned, this leads to chin and submental-cervical soft tissue ptosis [28]. For this reason, we avoid wide muscular detachment. No infection, bone reabsorption, or fixation instability were found in our patients, as have been reported in some series.

CONCLUSIONS

Surgical and non-surgical profileplasty are both fundamental techniques with various degrees of invasiveness—negligible in non-surgical and mini-invasive or clearly invasive in surgical, including also open rhinoplasty. The collective aim of these practices is to achieve a thorough full-like appearance of the facial profile, including specific Arnett's parameters and different ratios among the various facial areas in accordance with aging, ethnicity, and cultural tenets, with the simple yet complex purpose of obtaining a beautiful face. Harmonic proportions consider the fundamental anatomic parts contributing to the facial look, and the nose is probably the most crucial of these. This is a major reason to consider rhinoplasty in a deeper way, in both its non-surgical and its surgical approaches, as a fundamental item in aesthetic and rejuvenation medicine.

BIBLIOGRAPHY

1. Perkins SW. Modern facial profileplasty. Facial Plast Surg. 2019 Oct;35(5):421–422.
2. Pascali M, Marchese G, Diaspro A. The rhino-lip-lifting: a novel proposal for midface profileplasty performed as a single surgical procedure. Facial Plast Surg. 2021 Jun;37(3):340–347.
3. Bertossi D, Lanaro L, Dell'Acqua I, et al. Injectable profiloplasty: forehead, nose, lips, and chin filler treatment. J Cosmet Dermatol. 2019 Aug;18(4):976–984.
4. Nocini PF. Aesthetic improvements in mid-lower face skeletal surgery. Facial Plast Surg. 1999;15(4):285–296.
5. Farkas LG, Kolar JC. Anthropometrics and art in the aesthetics of women's faces. Clin Plast Surg. 1987 Oct;14(4):599–616.
6. Hönn M, Göz G. The ideal of facial beauty: a review. J Orofac Orthop. 2007 Jan;68(1):6–16. English, German. doi: 10.1007/s00056-007-0604-6.
7. Romeo F. Profiloplasty in one session versus single treatment areas. Dermatol Surg. 2021 Jul 1;47(7):953–958.
8. Buck DW 2nd, Alam M, Kim JY. Injectable fillers for facial rejuvenation: a review. J Plast Reconstr Aesthet Surg. 2009 Jan;62(1):11–18.
9. Bass LS. Injectable filler techniques for facial rejuvenation, volumization, and augmentation. Facial Plast Surg Clin North Am. 2015 Nov;23(4):479–488.
10. Chen HH, Williams EF. Lipotransfer in the upper third of the face. Curr Opin Otolaryngol Head Neck Surg. 2011 Aug;19(4):289–294.
11. Lee JH, Choi MS, Kim YH. Correction of deep static glabellar lines with acellular dermal matrix insertion. Ann Plast Surg. 2014 Dec;73(6):627–630.
12. Hotta TA. Understanding the anatomy of the upper face when providing aesthetic injection treatments. Plast Surg Nurs. 2016 Jul–Sep;36(3):104–109.

13. Jasin ME. Nonsurgical rhinoplasty using dermal fillers. Facial Plast Surg Clin North Am. 2013 May;21(2):241–252.
14. Moon HJ. Use of fillers in rhinoplasty. Clin Plast Surg. 2016 Jan;43(1):307–317.
15. Thomas WW, Bucky L, Friedman O. Injectables in the nose: facts and controversies. Facial Plast Surg Clin North Am. 2016 Aug;24(3):379–389.
16. Rauso R, Colella G, Zerbinati N, Salti G. Safety and early satisfaction assessment of patients seeking nonsurgical rhinoplasty with filler. J Cutan Aesthet Surg. 2017 Oct–Dec;10(4):207–214.
17. Solomon P, Sklar M, Zener R. Facial soft tissue augmentation with Artecoll(®): a review of eight years of clinical experience in 153 patients. Can J Plast Surg. 2012 Spring;20(1):28–32.
18. Lundström A, Lundström F, Lebret LM, Moorrees CF. Natural head position and natural head orientation: basic considerations in cephalometric analysis and research. Eur J Orthod. 1995 Apr;17(2):111–120.
19. Ricketts RM. Esthetics, environment, and the law of lip relation. Am J Orthod. 1968 Apr;54(4):272–289.
20. Merrifield LL. The profile line as an aid in critically evaluating facial esthetics. Am J Orthod. 1966 Nov;52(11):804–822.
21. Scheideman GB, Bell WH, Legan HL, et al. Cephalometric analysis of dentofacial normals. Am J Orthod. 1980 Oct;78(4):404–420.
22. Burstone CJ. Lip posture and its significance in treatment planning. Am J Orthod. 1967 Apr;53(4):262–284.
23. Edwards RC, Kiely KD, Eppley BL. Resorbable fixation techniques for genioplasty. J Oral Maxillofac Surg. 2000 Mar;58(3):269–272.
24. Segner D, Höltje WJ. Langzeitergebnisse nach Genioplastik [Long-term results after genioplasty]. Fortschr Kieferorthop. 1991 Oct;52(5):282–288.
25. Dann JJ, Epker BN. Proplast genioplasty: a retrospective study with treatment recommendations. Angle Orthod. 1977 Jul;47(3):173–185.
26. Bertossi D, Albanese M, Turra M, et al. Combined rhinoplasty and genioplasty: long-term follow-up. JAMA Facial Plast Surg. 2013 May;15(3):192–197.
27. McCarthy JG, Ruff GL, Zide BM. A surgical system for the correction of bony chin deformity. Clin Plast Surg. 1991 Jan;18(1):139–152.
28. Chaushu G, Blinder D, Taicher S, Chaushu S. The effect of precise reattachment of the mentalis muscle on the soft tissue response to genioplasty. J Oral Maxillofac Surg. 2001 May;59(5):510–516; discussion 517.

CHAPTER 9

Complications from Hyaluronic Acid Fillers

Koenraad De Boulle

A multitude of soft tissue fillers are currently available for facial aesthetic indications, ranging from autologous fat, polymethylmethacrylate, calcium hydroxyapatite, poly-L-lactic acid, polycaprolactone, and hyaluronic acid (HA) [1–5]. Because HA fillers have the powerful advantage of being completely removable using hyaluronidase (depending on approval in specific countries), they are referred to as reversible and are currently the most widely used dermal fillers. For this reason, this chapter is aimed primarily at complications arising from the use of HA fillers.

HA fillers currently constitute the second most performed aesthetic modality after botulinum toxin [1]. The tremendous market expansion, coupled with new treatment paradigms and inadequate control of both products and injectors, has heralded a concerning increase in serious adverse events [2,3]. Complication recognition and management have become the most significant unmet needs for filler treatments [4,5]. In addition, the use of injectable fillers has increased its popularity as an alternative to facial cosmetic surgery, as reported by the International Society of Aesthetic Plastic Surgery [6]. Filler injections allow physicians to obtain excellent results owing to their relatively easy nonsurgical delivery, rapid results, and low-cost office-based procedure. Surgical rhinoplasty, according to American Society of Aesthetic Plastic Surgery (ASAPS) statistics [7], is the sixth most requested procedure; however, nonsurgical rhinoplasty with fillers in the last few years has shown itself to be an effective alternative for patients who are looking for an aesthetic improvement of the nose. Fillers can sculpt the nasal shape by injections in the space between the skin and nasal skeleton, and this technique, called "nonsurgical rhinoplasty," has grown up during these years because their effects are visible immediately after treatment and patients can return to their normal activities on the same day.

Although fillers generally are considered safe, complications may occur, including immunoreactions, infections and cellulitis, skin necrosis, granuloma formation (a histologic diagnosis), and more severe adverse reactions such as ophthalmic and retinal artery occlusion or embolization [4]. The optimal approach to filler complications lies in having practical strategies for their prevention, as well as the insightful knowledge required for timely diagnosis and treatment.

Understanding the basic anatomical knowledge of the midface, especially the vascular system, is fundamental to reduce the risk of developing complications during nasal cosmetic injections. This chapter focuses on the main complications associated with nonsurgical rhinoplasty procedures, performed as injections of fillers (specifically HA), and on their management.

PREVENTION

All injectors should work with an operative strategy aimed at reducing the risk of complications. A number of issues need to be considered before engaging in treating patients with HA and, by extension, when performing non-surgical rhinoplasty.

1. **History and selection:** It is necessary to invest time in a pretreatment consultation, taking notes of skin conditions, systemic disease, medications, and previous procedures. Knowledge of previous surgical and nonsurgical cosmetic procedures is vital, as these could cause anatomical repositioning of structures and fixation and scarring of underlying vasculature, thus facilitating intravascular placement. Knowledge of the type and location of previously injected products may help to prevent compatibility issues with minimally degradable fillers [5]. The treatment plan should ideally be structured over time with due consideration given to pending medical procedures, dental visits, and immunizations. These steps aim to limit inflammatory reactions or hypersensitivities due to a heightened immune system.

    Skin barrier disruption due to inflammatory or infective conditions may persist for 3–4 weeks. Acne, rosacea, and dermatitis should be adequately considered, with 3–4 weeks' repair of optimal barrier function before filler treatments are performed [4]. Increased numbers of resistant *Propionibacterium acnes* at the edges of topically treated acne areas are thought to play a role in the formation of biofilms via the toll-like receptors (TLR-2), and the "safe distance" for filler placement relative to an area of acne is unknown. It is preferable to avoid injecting patients with multiple severe allergies and a history of anaphylaxis. Filler treatments have been contraindicated in active autoimmune diseases such as systemic lupus erythematosus, rheumatoid arthritis, and mixed connective tissue disease, but even in cases with longer follow-up, no disease exacerbation or reactivation was seen. Fillers seem to be more efficacious and safer to incorporate during quiescent stages of these diseases, but more trials are needed. A meta-analysis of all published cases in this field advised that for morphea and systemic sclerosis, skin fibrosis may create initial difficulties but appears to improve with subsequent sessions. Disease reactivation is not documented because all described cases had inactive disease. For lupus erythematosus (cutaneous and systemic), a theoretical risk of disease reactivation after tissue stimulation exists, but to date there are no literature reports [8–10].

Ascertain the current use of antibiotics and the indications thereof, as patients with remote infections involving the urinary tract, sinuses, intestinal tract, and oral cavity are best deferred for treatment. The hematogenous spread of normally non-virulent bacteria may lead to binding to the TLRs, with possible triggering of an immune response and formation of late-onset nodules many months later. Prophylactic antivirals are advised to prevent virus reactivation if there is a history of herpes simplex infection in the intended area of injection. Dental procedures, visits to the oral hygienist, and tooth bleaching/whitening are best avoided during the 2- to 4-week period before and after filler treatment to reduce the risk of hematogenous bacterial seeding and the potential development of biofilm [4].

2. **Insightful knowledge of injection anatomy** is of paramount importance in avoiding danger areas and serves as the foundation for avoiding disastrous complications. Although the exact position of vessels is highly variable, the plane in which they run is far more predictable. Therefore, knowledge of "safety by depth and location of danger areas" is a vital safety tool, as is constant awareness of the early signs of vascular compromise (Figures 9.1 and 9.2) [5]. Seckel has divided the face into seven danger zones, knowledge of which is important when treating specific regions [11], and they are in different areas where we can identify important vessels and nerves which may be involved during our injections [11]. For rhinoplasty the important zone is zone number 5: this zone lies at the superior orbital rim above the midpupil where the **supraorbital (cranial nerve [CN] V)** and the

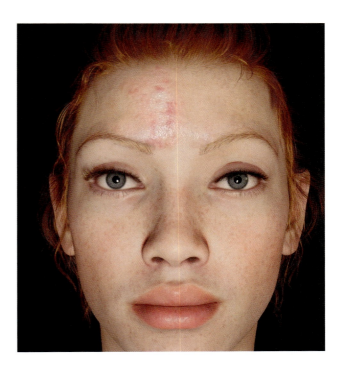

Figure 9.1 Compromised supratrochlear artery and/or vein.

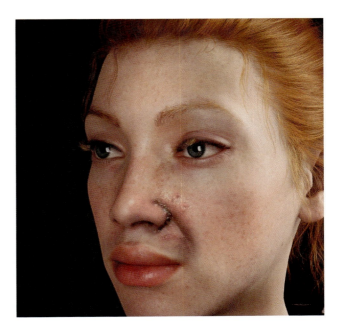

Figure 9.2 Compromised artery and/or angular vein.

more **medial supratrochlear (CN V) neurovascular bundles** are found. The supraorbital nerve (2.5 cm lateral to the midline), easily palpated at the supraorbital rim at the midpupil level, lies deep to the corrugator supercilii muscle (CSM), and the supratrochlear nerve (1.5 cm lateral to the midline) passes through the CSM. Nerve injury may cause numbness of the scalp, forehead, upper eyelid, and nasal dorsum, but intravascular injection during nasal injections (external carotid system) may cause blindness due to central retinal occlusion (CRO), since this artery is a terminal branch of the ophthalmic artery (internal carotid system), which communicates through the dorsal nasal arteries (Figure 9.3).

3. **Assessment:** Ethnicity, gender, and clinical needs are important to construct an applicable treatment plan. Specific measures in addressing, assessing, and understanding specific needs of individuals pertaining to the group of patients need to be applied [12–14].

4. **Informed consent:** Signed informed consent is crucial in creating awareness of the potential risk of filler-induced complications. It is wise to obtain informed consent for both the procedure and the management of inadvertent complications, should they arise, to expedite efficient management. This includes the discussion of possible, albeit rare, ophthalmic complications. Postprocedural instructions may include the injector/clinic being available via phone for 48 hours postprocedure (hence, contact numbers need to be handed out) and commonsense advice such as washing the face with uncontaminated water and using only new or unopened canisters or tubes with cosmetics for the first 24 hours [4]. It is good practice to have a staff member call the patient the next day. These instructions help to establish realistic expectations and minimize legal repercussions.

5. **Reversibility** is a powerful advantage when using HA products. Practical knowledge pertaining to locally available hyaluronidases and their effect on locally available HA fillers is of paramount importance, as the required dosages may differ. Certain products may require a higher dose of or more frequent injections with hyaluronidase. Additionally, when fibrosis is present after a certain period, the use of intralesional steroids might be necessary [4].

6. **Product characteristics** such as HA concentration and proprietary crosslinking should be understood in the context of ideal depth, placement, and duration. The hygroscopic nature of HA is an important determinant of product-related swelling and needs to be differentiated from procedural swelling. The HA concentration and extent of crosslinking determine the product's characteristics (viscosity, elasticity, resistance to degradation, G' [elastic modulus], G'' [viscous modulus], and tau delta), and ultimately its clinical efficacy and ideal depth of placement. Nasal injections must be done with very high G' HA [15–16].

7. **Product layering** over late or minimally degradable fillers is discouraged, and although HAs remain the most compatible fillers, it is wise to be cautious when considering cross-brand layering. Late or minimally biodegradable fillers may be provoked into reactivity when a second filler such as HA is layered over them, potentially inducing long-lasting complications such as biofilm formation or foreign body granulomas. Accurate records of the type and location of previously injected products may help to prevent compatibility issues with late or minimally degradable fillers, and the brand and type of the filler, as well as

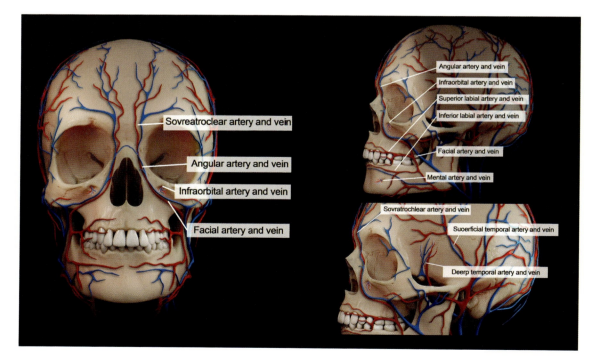

Figure 9.3 Intravascular injection risk zones.

the injected quantities, should be meticulously documented after each treatment [5].
8. **Photographic and video documentation** (pre- and postprocedure) is vital for patient monitoring, medio-legal purposes, and as a tool for self-education [4].
9. **Procedural planning and aseptic technique** are pivotal in avoiding complications, and it is essential to prevent breaching of the clean workspace. Makeup should be removed, and the skin cleansed carefully. Chlorhexidine antiseptic solutions are highly effective. However, they pose a risk to the middle ear and have the potential to irreversibly damage the cornea with a minimal splash exposure. An alternative might be, e.g., hypochlorous acid—a neutral superoxidase agent, safe around eyes and ears, and highly effective against *Staphylococcus aureus*, *Pseudomonas*, and *Escherichia coli* and also antifungal [17–18].

Consider the Following

a) The treating physician should remove all jewelry, wash their hands with antiseptic cleanser, and use gloves for all cases of injection therapy. The procedure is not deemed sterile, as the syringe itself is not completely sterile. Thus, sterility is lost once the syringe is handled, making aseptic technique of paramount importance [19]. Surgical principles of sterile technique—not touching any component of the needle or cannula that penetrates the skin—may further reduce infective complications.
b) Stringent aseptic technique is mandatory: cleanse, degrease, and disinfect. There are no universally recommended topical antiseptics, but chlorhexidine, chloroxylenol, iodophors, alcohol, iodine, and hypochlorous acid may be appropriate.
c) Have everything at hand to reduce breaks in the aseptic field and the concomitant risk of injection-related infections.
d) Rinsing the mouth with an antiseptic mouthwash containing chlorhexidine (0.2%) or iodine-povidone [20] adequately disinfects the oral cavity for up to 8 hours and has been suggested as a preventative practice for perioral treatments or patients with a lip-licking habit.
e) Frequent needle (and cannula) changes are advised for multiple entry points.

10. **Technical knowledge** of placement and injection depth is cardinal to the success of dermal fillers.

Strategies for optimizing technique include:

- Knowledge of injection anatomy.
- Awareness of danger areas.
- Aspiration before injecting where applicable.
- Slow injection speed with the least amount of pressure possible.
- Moving tip with delivery of product where applicable.
- Incrementally injecting small 0.1–0.2 mL aliquots of product.
- Use of a small syringe to deliver precise aliquots.
- Use of a small needle to slow down injection speed.
- Use of a blunt cannula where indicated.
- Careful consideration of the patient's medical history.
- Stopping injection if resistance is encountered or the patient experiences pain/discomfort.
- It is vital to routinely check perfusion in the treated areas, as well as areas with watershed perfusion (glabella, nasal tip, upper lip), ensuring that makeup is not obscuring skin tone.
- Initial signs of vascular compromise may be subtle and fleeting.

CLASSIFICATION OF COMPLICATIONS FROM HYALURONIC ACID FILLERS

The literature [4,21–24] currently classifies complications based on the *time of onset*, dividing them into immediate, early, and late-onset complications:

- **Immediate complications** (within 24 hours): Bruising or hematoma, swelling, erythema, reactivation of a herpes infection, bacterial infection, nodules from product accumulation, pain, immediate type I allergic reaction, paresthesia, Tyndall effect, improper filler placement, or vascular complications. These are usually the easiest to manage, except for the vascular ones that are far more serious, representing an absolute urgent situation and can lead to significant therapeutic difficulties.
- **Early complications** (within 4 weeks): Nodules due to misplacement or migration of the filler, hematomas, reactivation of a herpetic infection, bacterial infection, type I hypersensitivity, Tyndall effect, or paresthesia.
- **Late complications** (more than 4 weeks): Non-inflammatory nodules (see early complications) or inflammatory nodules (Figures 9.4 and 9.5), which are subdivided into single or multifocal (including granulomas) resulting from late bacterial infections, generally mediated by biofilms, infections caused by atypical mycobacteria, cyclic edema of inflammatory nature, or the Tyndall effect.

Another approach to classification of the most common complications from HA fillers can be based on the *severity of the complications* themselves, according to the following definitions and scheme:

- **Complications of a mild degree**: Generally with immediate onset, which resolve spontaneously in 24–48 hours without sequelae.
- **Moderate-degree complications**: They can be early or late, with their resolution requiring intervention by the specialist and the administration of appropriate therapy.
- **Severe complications**: May be either early or late, requiring a timely intervention by the specialist (vascular complications); they can leave permanent signs (visual impairment, necrosis, scars).

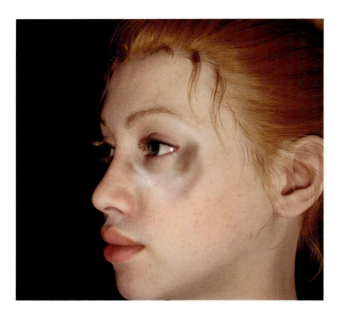

Figure 9.4 Late nodule in the tear trough (courtesy of Dr. Gloria Trocchi).

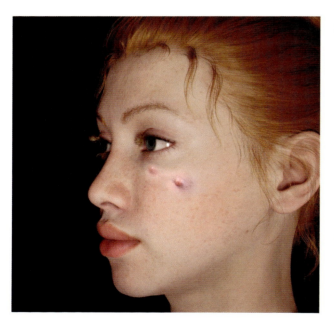

Figure 9.5 Late nodules in the malar area (courtesy of Dr. Gloria Trocchi).

DIAGNOSIS, PREVENTION, AND THERAPY OF SEVERE COMPLICATIONS FROM HYALURONIC ACID FILLERS

Vascular Complications

Vascular complications occur because of accidental direct injection of the filler into a vessel resulting in embolization in the surrounding areas, but also in distant locations (upstream and downstream) [25, 26]. They are usually of immediate onset and can cause very significant damage, possibly of even dramatic proportions, up to the necrosis of the tissues supplied by the occluded vessel or loss of vision. The cases described in the literature are now anything but rare, and it is believed that the real incidence of these complications is underestimated.

Diagnosis and Symptoms

Rapid dyschromia, or whitening in the metameric vascular territory, depending on the area of injection, followed by reticular livedo and herpes simplex–like vesicle and pustule formation, can occur in the following days. Occasionally, the patient may complain of pain, but this is not a consistent diagnostic sign. Such symptoms do not necessarily occur in a fixed order and may occur even in the very first days after treatment. Therefore, it is important to instruct the patient to promptly inform the physician of any changes in skin color in the treated areas in the days following the treatment session [4].

Prevention of Vascular Complications

Extreme care must be taken in areas of high vascular risk, injecting slowly, at the correct depth, and avoiding excessive amounts of product per injection site; moreover, aspiration before injection, especially in the most critical areas, is recommended by many to avoid vascular risk [27], although the perception of safety derived from aspiration is now the subject of debate [28,29].

For the nasal area in particular, pay attention to dorsal and external nasal arteries and veins and to lateral nasal artery, and for the nasolabial folds pay attention to the facial artery and vein and nasal branches.

Treatment of Vascular Complications

Nowadays the protocol described by De Lorenzi [30] aims to dissolve the obstruction (or compression) by flushing the tissues with hyaluronidase. As simple clinical observation does not allow the physician to understand how much material has entered the vascular tree or to identify the precise location of the obstruction, it is necessary to repeatedly inject high doses of hyaluronidase over the entire affected area—called "flooding the area with hyaluronidase".

This protocol for "high-dose pulsed hyaluronidase" (HDPH) is suggested, which consists of the repeated administration of high doses of hyaluronidase throughout the area affected by ischemia. The protocol assumes that, in the case of filler embolization, all vessels in the affected area are obstructed. To obtain an effective concentration of hyaluronidase per cc in a given area of the face, a high quantity of

Table 9.1 HDPH Treatment Protocol Proposed by C. De Lorenzi [30] for the Treatment of Vascular Complications from Hyaluronic Acid Filler

HDPH (high dose pulsed hyaluronidase) protocol	
Affected Areas of the Face	Quantity of Hyaluronidase (IU)
One single area	500
Two areas of the face	1000
Three or more areas of the face	≥1500

Note: Treatment should be repeated every hour until signs of ischemia have completely resolved, so as to ensure that optimal vascularization of the embolized area is restored.

hyaluronidase must therefore be injected. The hourly rate of infiltration is a substantial aspect of the protocol because the frequent administration compensates for the rapid deactivation and dilution of hyaluronidase. Repeated treatment every hour ensures that a high concentration of active hyaluronidase is maintained in the perivascular tissues and therefore, due to high diffusion through the vessel wall, even within the lumen of the affected vessels. It is essential to remember, in fact, that only hyaluronidase that manages to penetrate inside the vessels is effective in determining the breakdown of intravascular HA. The dosage suggested by De Lorenzi is 500 IU if the ischemic area involves a single area of the face (e.g., lip or glabellar region), 1000 IU if it involves two areas of the face (e.g., lip and nose), and up to over 1500 IU if three or more areas are involved (Table 9.1) [30]. According to the HDPH protocol, treatment ends when signs of ischemia have been completely resolved so as to ensure the restoration of an optimal vascularization of the affected area. This is easily ascertained by compressing the affected area and assessing the capillary filling time at release.

The enzyme can diffuse through the vascular walls and induce lysis of the obstructions caused by HA [30]. In contrast, attempting to penetrate the occluded vessel with precision is illusory, unless massive doses of hyaluronidase are injected upstream in easily accessible points, like the arteria facialis at the mandibular border or other areas visible with ultrasound [31].

Also worth mentioning is that hyaluronidase injections are worthless after 3–4 days after the incident. Hyaluronidase cannot permeate thrombotic masses, inherently formed in front of the hygroscopic bolus of HA, blocking the vessel due to platelet aggregation.

Late Occurring Reactions

In general these complications can occur from 4–6 weeks to a year or more after treatment and they are generally of an inflammatory nature.

Diagnosis and Symptoms

Delayed inflammatory reactions (DIRs) secondary to tissue filler administration develop after at least 2–4 weeks or later following an HA injection. The clinical manifestations occur in the form of recurrent episodes of localized solid edema with erythema and tenderness or as subcutaneous nodules at the site of HA injection.

In recent years the literature has also highlighted the role of biofilm in the genesis of late chronic complications of these materials [32]. The bacteria that will give rise to biofilm can penetrate along with the filler if the rules of asepsis are not correctly implemented by the injecting physician, hence their prevention-oriented importance. As these are low-grade contaminations, it may take months before they become clinically manifest.

However, the development of inflammatory nodules in areas located at some distance from the site of injection, resistance of the lesion to long-lasting antibiotic treatment, and the exclusion of an infectious agent (cultures and polymerase chain reaction [PCR] test) raise doubts about the role of biofilm. Moreover, the effectiveness of treatment with hyaluronidase and the dependence on the volume of HA administered suggest the mechanism of delayed hypersensitivity [33].

Aside from biofilm formation, other pathogenetic causes must be considered. Filler characteristics (degree of crosslinking, concentration of HA) and host characteristics (local and systemic) may play a role. Non-specific immune reactions, specifically type I and type IV hypersensitivity, and an adjuvant role of hyaluronic acid (autoimmune/inflammatory syndrome induced by adjuvants [ASIA] syndrome) may all contribute to the genesis of DIRs [34].

Late chronic inflammatory complications may also occur shortly after episodes of bacteremia (dental treatment, urinary infections, skin abscesses, etc.), showing that the bacteria forming a biofilm in the proximity of the filler can reach it from distant locations many months after the treatment session.

Viral infections (flulike disease and COVID-19) [35,36] are known to be able to elicit a late inflammatory reaction to the filler.

Treatment

From a therapeutic point of view, the drugs used in these situations are corticosteroids, hyaluronidase, and antibiotics. The problem resides in establishing their sequence and dosage.

The most recent literature, which has strongly emphasized the role of biofilm, tends to favor immediate high-dose antibiotics [4,5,21,24,33]. Corticosteroids are not to be considered first-line drugs in the management of these complications, as they are essentially infectious [37,38]. However, the contribution of corticosteroids as antiinflammatory and immunomodulators cannot be ignored and do certainly have a place in the therapeutic approach of DIRs.

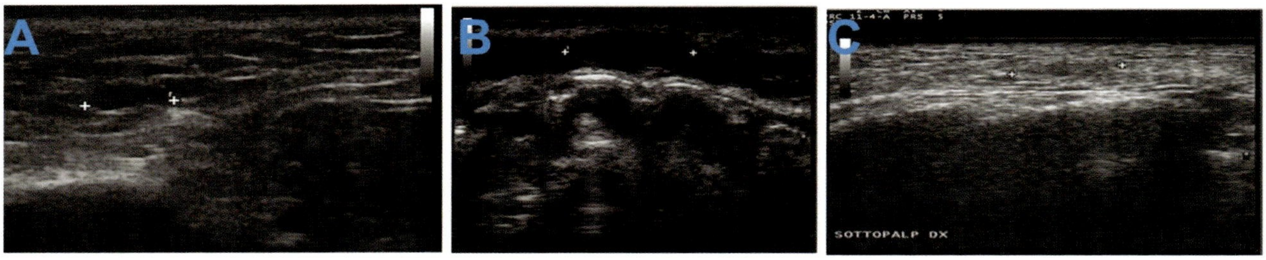

Figure 9.6 A) Presence of anechoic collections in the dermis; B) accumulation of hyaluronic acid in the labial area; C) nodules and edema with a tendency to fibrosis (courtesy of Dr. Rita Cammarata).

Clinicians have generally always avoided administering corticosteroids in case of active infections because of their known immunosuppressive effects and possible long-term side effects. However, there is now scientific evidence of the efficacy and safety of corticosteroids in several bacterial infections [39,40], even in biofilm infections; in vitro studies have demonstrated a direct antibacterial effect against biofilm infections [41].

A viable protocol might be simultaneous treatment with antibiotics and corticosteroids for the first week, then continuing with tapering down the steroids and continuing the antibiotic therapy alone for a total of 2–4 weeks. The use of hyaluronidase is possibly reserved for a second therapeutic phase in case this first phase yields insufficient results.

Hyaluronidase injections in the treatment of DIR may be effective in removing the inflamed HA filler, but only needs to be considered in the final stage, after all other options are tried out, as removing the filler will simultaneously and inevitably also remove the aesthetic improvement achieved [42].

For long-standing nodules, where a certain degree of fibrosis is present, repeated intralesional injection with corticosteroids, eventually combined with 5-fluorouracil, might be of benefit [4,42].

Contribution of Imaging

The support of an ultrasound examination, a non-invasive technique that doesn't use an x-ray, can be helpful in identifying the type of material. In addition, it allows the identification of the material that infiltrated according to its ultrasound image: anechoic, hyperechoic, or hypoechoic. The presence of well-defined and delimited anechoic deposits is characteristic of HA accumulations (Figure 9.6) [43,44].

CONCLUSIONS

Prevention is not only essential but possible. Professional medical training and accurate medical history taking can prevent a considerable number of complications.

Vascular occlusion is always an emergency and needs to be approached adequately and aggressively with hyaluronidase. Delayed inflammatory reactions are bothersome, but treatment protocols based on oral antibiotics, eventually oral steroids, and in the last resort hyaluronidase have proven to be effective.

BIBLIOGRAPHY

1. Carruthers J, Carruthers A, Tezel A, et al. Volumizing with a 20-mg/mL smooth, highly cohesive, viscous hyaluronic acid filler and its role in facial rejuvenation therapy. Dermatol Surg. 2010;36(Suppl 3):1886–1892.
2. Goldberg RA, Fiaschetti D. Filling the periorbital hollows with hyaluronic acid gel: initial experience with 244 injections. Ophthal Plast Reconstr Surg 2006;22:335–341.
3. Callan P, Goodman GJ, Carlisle I, et al. Efficacy and safety of a hyaluronic acid filler in subjects treated for correction of midface volume deficiency: a 24-months study. Clin Cosmet Investig Dermatol. 2013;6:81–89.
4. Heydenrych I, De Boulle K, Kapoor KM, Bertossi D. The 10-point plan 2021: updated concepts for improved procedural safety during facial filler treatments. Clin Cosmet Investig Dermatol. 2021 Jul 6;14:779–814.
5. De Boulle K, Heydenrych I. Patient factors influencing dermal filler complications: prevention, assessment, and treatment. Clin Cosmet Investig Dermatol. 2015;8:205–214.
6. International Society of Aesthetic Plastic Surgery. ISAPS global statistics. June 2022. Available at: www.isaps.org/medical-professionals/isaps-global-statistics/.
7. American Society for Aesthetic Plastic Surgery. Cosmetic surgery national data bank statistics. June 2022. Available at: www.surgery.org/sites/default/files/ASAPS-Stats2016.pdf.
8. Gonzalez C, Pamatmat J, Goff H. Safety and efficacy of dermal fillers in patients with connective tissue disease: a review. Dermatol Surg. 2021 Mar 1;47(3): 360–364.
9. Creadore A, et al. Cosmetic treatment in patients with autoimmune connective tissue diseases: best practices for patients with morphea/systemic sclerosis. J Am Acad Dermatol. 2020 Aug;83(2):315–341.

10. Creadore A, et al. Cosmetic treatment in patients with autoimmune connective tissue diseases: best practices for patients with lupus erythematosus. J Am Acad Dermatol. 2020 Aug;83(2):343–363.
11. Seckel B. Facial danger zones: avoiding nerve injury in facial plastic surgery. Thieme; 2010, pp. 1–49.
12. de Maio M. Ethnic and gender considerations in the use of facial injectables: male patients. Plast Reconstr Surg. 2015 Nov;136(5 Suppl):40S–43S.
13. De Boulle K, Furuyama N, Heydenrych I, et al. Considerations for the use of minimally invasive aesthetic procedures for facial remodeling in transgender individuals. Clin Cosmet Investig Dermatol. 2021 May 13;14:513–525.
14. Sundaram H, Liew S, Signorini M, et al. Global aesthetics consensus group: global aesthetics consensus: hyaluronic acid fillers and botulinum toxin type A-recommendations for combined treatment and optimizing outcomes in diverse patient populations. Plast Reconstr Surg. 2016 May;137(5):1410–1423.
15. Tezel A, Fredrickson G. The science of hyaluronic acid fillers. J Cosmet Laser Ther. 2008;10:35–42.
16. Micheels P, Eng MO. Rheological properties of several hyaluronic acid–based gels: a comparative study. J Drugs Dermatol. 2018;17:948–954.
17. Steinsapir K. Chlorhexidine keratitis: safety of chlorhexidine as a facial antiseptic. Dermatol Surg. 2016;43(1).
18. Del Rosso J. Status report on topical hypochlorous acid. J Clin Aesthet Dermatol. 2018;11:36–39.
19. Rowley S, Clare S. ANTT: a standard approach to aseptic technique. Nurs Times. 2011;19;107(36):12–14.
20. Kirk-Bayley J. The use of povidone iodine nasal spray and mouthwash during the current COVID-19 pandemic may protect healthcare workers and reduce cross infection. Available SSRN 3563092. 2020.
21. Heydenrych I, Kapoor KM, De Boulle K, et al. A 10-point plan for avoiding hyaluronic acid dermal filler-related complications during facial aesthetic procedures and algorithms for management. Clin Cosmet Investig Dermatol. 2018 Nov 23;11:603–611.
22. Signorini M, Liew S, Sundaram H, et al. Global aesthetics consensus: avoidance and management of complications from hyaluronic acid fillers-evidence and opinion-based review and consensus recommendations. Plast Reconstr Surg. 2016;137:961e–971e.
23. de Maio M, De Boulle K, Braz A, Rohrich RJ. Alliance for the future of aesthetics consensus committee: facial assessment and injection guide for botulinum toxin and injectable hyaluronic acid fillers: focus on the midface. Plast Reconstr Surg. 2017;140:540e–550e.
24. Philipp-Dormston WG, Goodman GJ, et al. Global approaches to the prevention and management of delayed-onset adverse reactions with hyaluronic acid–based fillers. Plast Reconstr Surg Glob Open. 2020 Apr 29;8(4):e2730.
25. Ashton M, Taylor I, Corlett R. The role of anastomotic vessels in controlling tissue viability and defining tissue necrosis with special reference to complications following injection of hyaluronic acid fillers. Plast Reconstr Surg. 2018 Jun;141(6):818e–830e.
26. De Lorenzi C. Complications of injectable fillers, part 2: vascular complications. Aesthet Surg J. 2014;34:584–600.
27. Tseng FW, Bommareddy K, Frank K, et al. Descriptive analysis of 213 positive blood aspiration cases when injecting facial soft tissue fillers. Aesthet Surg J. 2020. doi: 10.1093/asj/sjaa075.
28. Goodman et al. Neither positive nor negative aspiration before filler injection should be relied upon as a safety maneuver. Aesthet Surg J. Apr 2021;41(4).
29. Goodman GJ, Magnusson MR, Callan P, et al. Aspiration before tissue filler-an exercise in futility and unsafe practice. Aesthet Surg J. 2022 Jan 1;42(1):89–101.
30. DeLorenzi C. New high dose pulsed hyaluronidase protocol for hyaluronic acid filler vascular adverse events. Aesthet Surg J. 2017;37:814–825.
31. Lin F, Goodman GJ, Magnusson M, et al. Movement of the syringe during filler aspiration: an ultrasound study. Aesthet Surg J. 2022 Mar 26:sjac032.
32. Christensen LH. Host tissue interaction, fate, and risks of degradable and non-degradable gel fillers. Dermatol Surg. 2009;35:1612–1619.
33. Owczarczyk-Saczonek A, Zdanowska N, et al. The immunogenicity of hyaluronic fillers and its consequences. Clin Cosmet Investig Dermatol. 2021 Jul 16;14:921–934.
34. Alijotas-Reig J, Esteve-Valverde E, Gil-Aliberas N, Garcia-Gimenez V. Autoimmune/inflammatory syndrome induced by adjuvants-ASIA-related to biomaterials: analysis of 45 cases and comprehensive review of the literature et al. Immunol Res. 2018 Feb;66(1):120–140.
35. Turkmani MG, De Boulle K, Philipp-Dormston WG. Delayed hypersensitivity reaction to hyaluronic acid dermal filler following influenza-like illness. Clin Cosmet Investig Dermatol. 2019 Apr 29;12:277–283.
36. Munavalli G, Knutsen-Larson S, Lupo M, Geronemus R. Oral angiotensin converting enzyme inhibitors for the treatment of delayed inflammatory reaction of dermal hyaluronic acid fillers following COVID-19 vaccination—a model for inhibition of angiotensin ii-induced cutaneous inflammation. JAAD Case Rep. 2021;10:63–68.
37. de Maio M, Swift A, Signorini M, Fagien S. Aesthetic leaders in facial aesthetics consensus committee: facial assessment and injection guide for botulinum toxin and injectable hyaluronic acid fillers: focus on the upper face. Plast Reconstr Surg. 2017;140:265e–276e.
38. de Maio M, DeBoulle K, Braz A, Rohrich RJ. Alliance for the future of aesthetics consensus committee: facial assessment and injection guide for botulinum toxin and injectable hyaluronic acid fillers: focus on the midface. Plast Reconstr Surg. 2017;140:540e–550e.
39. McGee S. Use of corticosteroids in treating infectious diseases. Arch Intern Med. 2008;168:1034–1046.
40. Pereira JM, Lisboa T, Paiva JA. Adjuvant therapies in critical care: steroids to treat infectious diseases. Intensive Care Med. 2018;44:1306–1309.

41. Goggin A. Corticosteroids directly reduce staphylococcus aureus biofilm growth: An in vitro study. Laryngoscope. 2014;124:602–607.
42. Snozzi P, van Loghem JAJ. Complication management following rejuvenation procedures with hyaluronic acid fillers an algorithm-based approach. Plast Reconstr Surg Glob Open. 2018;6:e2061.
43. Schelke LW, Decates TS, Velthuis PJ. Ultrasound to improve the safety of hyaluronic acid filler treatments. J Cosmet Dermatol. 2018 Dec;17(6):1019–1024.
44. Schelke LW, Cassuto D, Velthuis P, Wortsman X. Nomenclature proposal for the sonographic description and reporting of soft tissue fillers. J Cosmet Dermatol. 2020 Feb;19(2):282–288.

CHAPTER **10**

Clinical Cases from the Experts

Introductory Video Section

Dario Bertossi

The videos cited throughout this text are available for those with the book to access at https://resourcecentre.routledge.com/books/9781032303444

Video 10.1	Overprojected nose and microgenia: Injections with very high G' filler
Video 10.2	Nasal hump and microgenia: Injections with very high G' filler
Video 10.3	Irregular nasal dorsum and microgenia: Injections with very high G' filler
Video 10.4	Nasal hump: Injections with very high G' filler
Video 10.5	Nasal hump: Injection with very high G' hyaluronic acid
Video 10.6	Retroprojected nasal base: Injections with very high G' filler
Video 10.7	Nasal hump: Injections with very high G' filler
Video 10.8	Nasal hump and microgenia: Injections with very high G' filler
Video 10.9	Very high G' filler
Video 10.10	Very high G' filler
Video 10.11	Very high G' filler

CHAPTER 10.1

Non-Surgical Rhinoplasty
Long-Term Correction after Five Years

Ada Trindade de Almeida

Nasal treatment with hyaluronic acid (HA) fillers is becoming a frequent aesthetic procedure because of its immediate result, no downtime and reversibility.

The nasal dorsum is a region of low movement, low shear stress, high compression, tight skin and muscle over bone structure [1]. In order to obtain and keep projection over time and to avoid lateral spread, the best choice is for HA fillers with high elasticity (capacity to recover its shape after deformation) and medium to high cohesivity (adhesion forces within the gel that make it stay together) [1].

The objective of this case is to demonstrate a long-lasting effect of non-surgical rhinoplasty with HA filler. A 24-year-old female asked for correction of a dropped nasal tip and dorsal hump (Figure 10.1.1). Voluma was chosen for its high elasticity and cohesivity and for its high lift capacity and relative longer duration (around 18 months) [2–3].

The patient received 0.1 mL at each of three sites: nasion, nasal dorsum and nasal tip and 0.25 mL in the right and left nasal bones (pyriform fossa) [4]. All areas were treated with a 27G needle through gentle and slow supraperiosteal injections (Figure 10.1.2).

Since she lives in another city, her follow-up visit was scheduled after 2 months, when a good result was confirmed with patient and physician satisfaction. She returned again after 5 years for new treatment that was not necessary because the aesthetic result was still present, particularly in the nasal tip and nasal dorsum (Figures 10.1.3–10.1.5).

Although HA fillers are expected to be reabsorbed, the longer duration in the nasal region may be explained

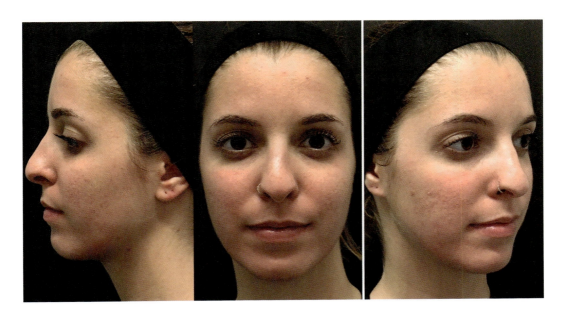

Figure 10.1.1   A 24-year-old patient with dropped nasal tip and nasal hump.

DOI: 10.1201/9781003304623-25

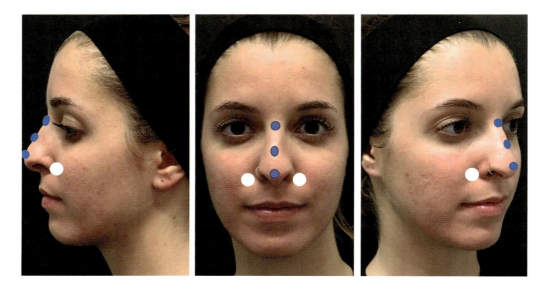

Figure 10.1.2 Treatment with Juvéderm Voluma: Blue circles = 0.1 mL each; nasal tip, nasal dorsum, nasium. White circles = 0.25 mL each. Total volume injected = 0.8 mL.

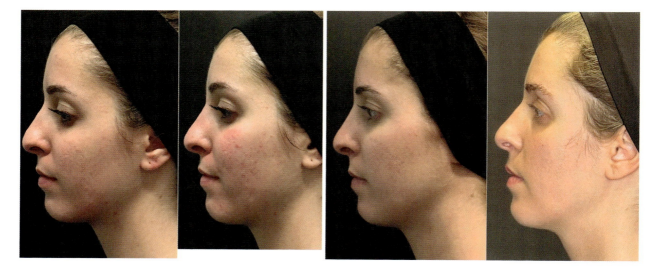

Figure 10.1.3 a and b Pre- and postoperative; c 2 months postoperative; d, 4 years 6 months postoperative.

LONG-TERM CORRECTION AFTER FIVE YEARS

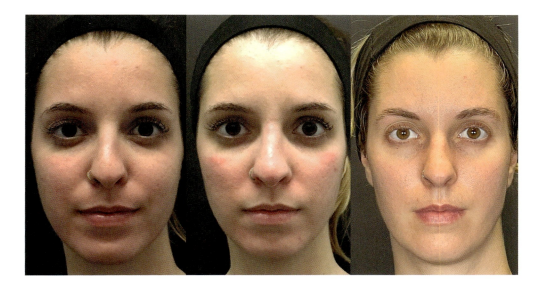

Figure 10.1.4 a and b Pre- and postoperative; c, 2 months postoperative; d, 4 years 6 months postoperative.

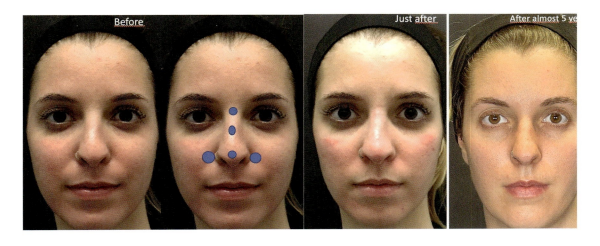

Figure 10.1.5 a and b Pre- and postoperative; c, 2 months postoperative; d, 4 years 6 months postoperative.

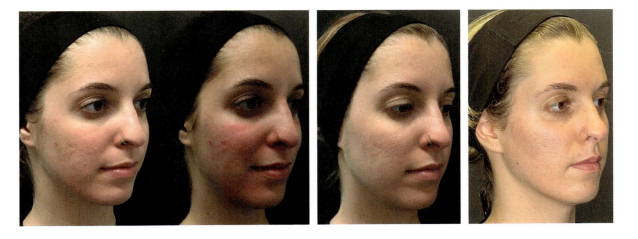

Figure 10.1.6

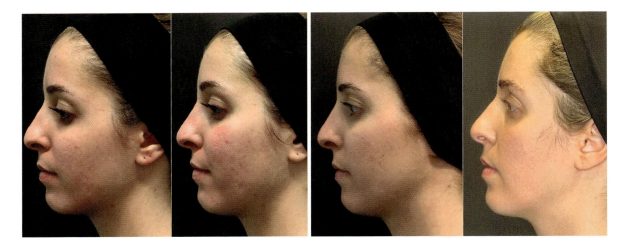

Figure 10.1.7

by the degree of cross-linking of the product, the paucity of local movements or even the partial replacement of the filler by new autologous tissue [5].

BIBLIOGRAPHY

1. La guardia C, Virno A, Musumeci M, Bernadim A, Silbeberg M. Rheologic and physicochemical characteristics of HA fillers: overview and relationship to product performance. Facial Plast Surg. 2022 Feb; 3. ahead of print.
2. Humphrey S, Carruthers J, Carruthers A. Clinical experience with 11,460 mL of a 20-mg/mL, smooth, highly cohesive, viscous hyaluronic acid filler. Dermatol Surg. 2015;41(9):1060–1067.
3. Goodman G, Swift A, Remington K. Current concepts in the use of Voluma, Volift and Volbella. Plast Reconstr Surg. 2015;136:139S–148S.
4. Bertossi D, Lanaro L, Dell'Acqua I, Albanese M, et al. Injectable profiloplasty: forehead, nose, lips and chin filler treatment. J Cosmet Dermatol. 2019;18(4):976–984.
5. Mochizuki M, Aoi N, Gonda K, Hirabayashi S, Komuro Y. Evaluation of the in vivo kinetics and biostimulatory effects of subcutaneously injected hyaluronic acid filler. Plast Reconstr Surg. 2018;142(1):112–121.

CHAPTER 10.2

Asian Cases

Chris Qiong Li

In terms of ethnic evolution, Asians often show brachycephalic head shapes, which indicate the head width is relatively larger in comparison to the length. Similarly, Asians possess relatively flat faces and sometimes typically flat noses. In some severe cases, the flat nose also is accompanied by a receding forehead, glabella area, low nasal bridge and even small chin.

Therefore, nose augmentations are a highly requested procedures in Asian countries. A lower nose and flat face is considered a sign of a lack of attractiveness, especially in the younger generations.

Existing techniques for rhinoplasty are using implants or autologous cartilage; however, most of the surgery is expensive and has a long recovery time and implant-related complications. Therefore, patients prefer not to undergo a surgical rhinoplasty. This has led to an increasing popularity of non-surgical rhinoplasty with fillers.

There are lots of products in the market, such as hyaluronic acid (HA), collagen, collagen-stimulator products, permanent fillers, etc. However, HA is still the dominant product for the non-surgical nose augmentation, mainly because it can last a longer time and is the only material that can be degraded with hyaluronidase, thereby minimizing the risk of filler-related vascular compromise. It is the same situation all over the world.

Patient selection is vital for satisfactory results. Not all patients who need rhinoplasty can be satisfied with filler augmentation. Only a mild to medium flat radix, dorsal hump, mildly deviated nose or slightly flat or downward-pointing nose tip can be the proper indication for filler nose augmentation. Severe problems (totally flat radix, huge dorsal hump, short nose, upturned nose tip or obvious deviated nose) and highly demanding patients should be excluded. In addition, caution is required when the patients have had a previous rhinoplasty (implant or autologous cartilage insertion) or liquid silicone injections, because there will be a much higher risk of skin irregularities and vascular compromise in those kinds of patients.

There are some tips for HA nose augmentation in the Asian population:

- Botulinum toxin injection can make the filler augmentation results much better because it can paralyze the muscles over the nose and prevent filler migration. It also can be helpful to improve dynamic nasal tip ptosis or alar flaring.
- Mainly, the non-surgical nose augmentation procedure with filler is classified into two parts: the dorsum of the nose and the tip of the nose. It is easier to lift up the upper part of the nose, while it is harder to lift or elongate the nasal tip, especially when patients have weak supporting structures.
- The midline should be marked before treatment to prevent imbalance deformity or intravascular injection (most of the vessels are not located in the midline of the nose).
- It is important to identify the nasal radix starting point for an optimal aesthetic result. Generally, the nasal radix begins at the level of the supratarsal fold in lateral view in Asians. Too high or too low a nasal radix will bring an odd look after the treatment and the patient might not be satisfied.
- A very high and wide nose bridge in Asian patients is not a good choice for physicians. The nose should be assessed not only as an individual facial unit but also should be considered as one part of the whole face. Most of the Asian faces do not possess a high frontal bone, especially prominent superciliary ridges; the nose height and width should be suitable with the total face. Otherwise, an avatar nose might be created.
- The nose tip injection weight is the same as with radix augmentation. Because some patients have a weak tip supporting structure and the tip is turning downward, tip columella and supratip area injection can ensure a better result and avoid the polybeak deformity.
- It is strongly recommended that the surgeon use two hands during the injection, one dominant hand for the injection, while the non-dominant hand lifts the skin and guides the needle into the tissue. In this way, it can minimize deformity and filler diffusion.

- The HA filler should be placed along the periosteum; this can minimize the intravascular injection because it is an avascular plane. Also, it can prevent the visibility of the filler after injection.
- A proper amount of HA injection is very important for both optimal results and safety. There will be a higher risk if too much filler is injected on the nose, especially on the tip of the nose, because the tissue space under the tight nose skin is so limited, and it can compromise blood supply by high tension.

See Figures 10.2.1 and 10.2.2.

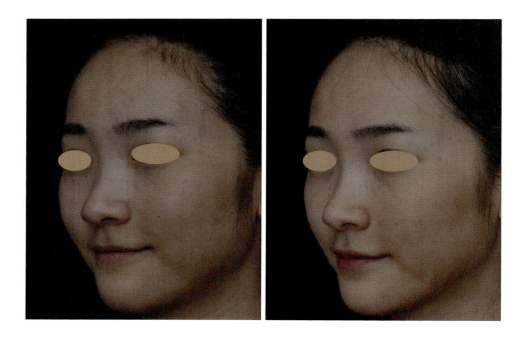

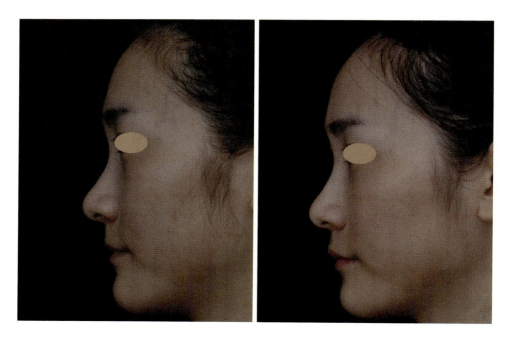

Figure 10.2.1a–d Female, 31 years old, non-surgical nose augmentation with HA filler, before and after.

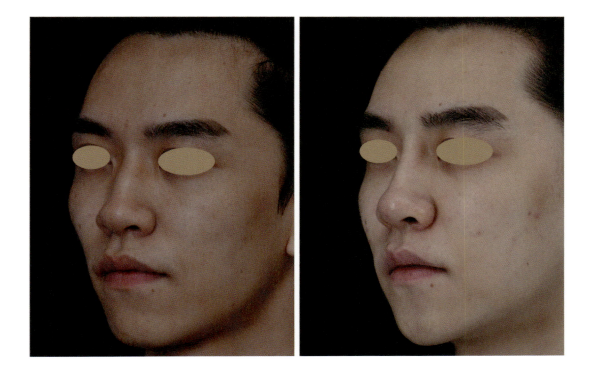

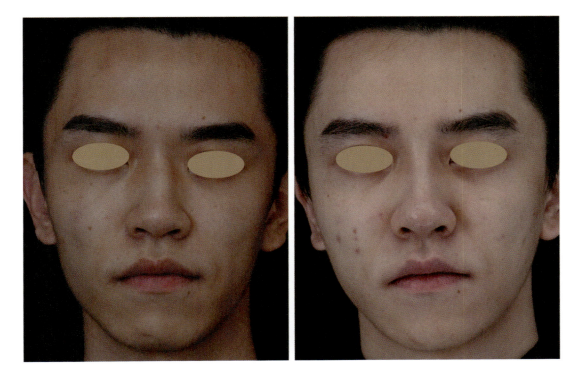

Figure 10.2.2a–d Male, 28 years old, non-surgical nose augmentation with HA filler (1.5 mL Perlane; injected to the root, dorsal and columella nasi; before and 1 week posttreatment).

CHAPTER **10.3**

Clinical Case
Profileplasty

Dario Bertossi

A female patient presented with an overprojected nasal tip, with a strong depressor septi nasi and thin skin, and also with microgenia. This is a classic clinical case of profileplasty. I inject such a patient on the nasal base (0.5 mL per side) and then on the anterior nasal spine (0.3 mL) with Volux (Allergan-Abbvie, USA), then on the infratip lobule (0.2 mL), as well as on the nasal tip between the domes (0.1 mL) and finally on the glabella (0.2 mL) and the nasal dorsum (0.2 mL). The chin is treated with 2 ml of Volux in the midline and along the anterior portion of the jawline. Finally, we inject Volift (1 mL) to reshape the lips. The result is good with no bruising and no pain (Figures 10.3.1–10.3.4).

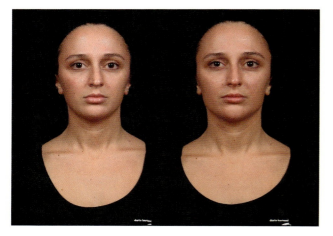
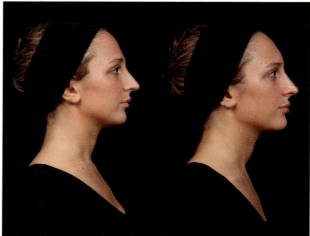
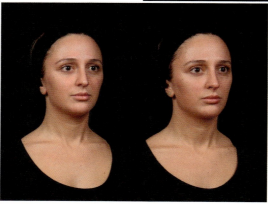

Figure 10.3.1 Patient 1: a, Frontal view, before and after; b, profile view, before and after; c, three-quarters view, before and after.

CLINICAL CASE: PROFILEPLASTY

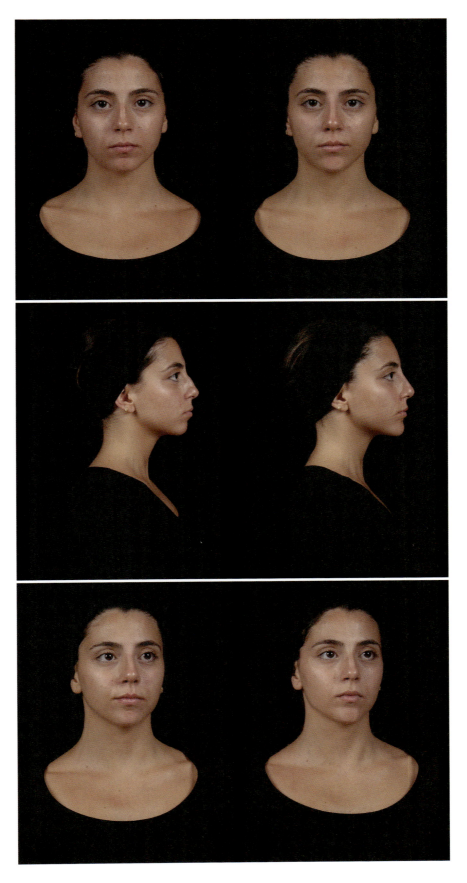

Figure 10.3.2 Patient 2: a, Frontal view, before and after; b, profile view, before and after; c, three-quarters view, before and after.

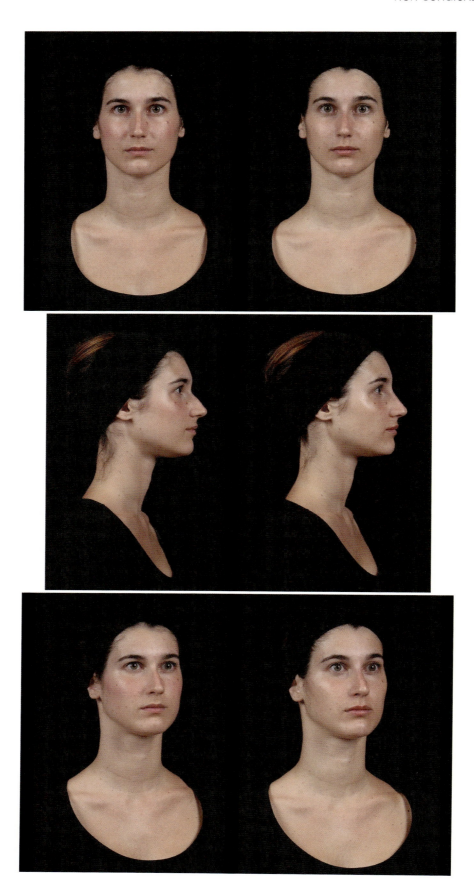

Figure 10.3.3 Patient 3: a, Frontal view, before and after; b, profile view, before and after; c, three-quarters view, before and after.

CLINICAL CASE: PROFILEPLASTY

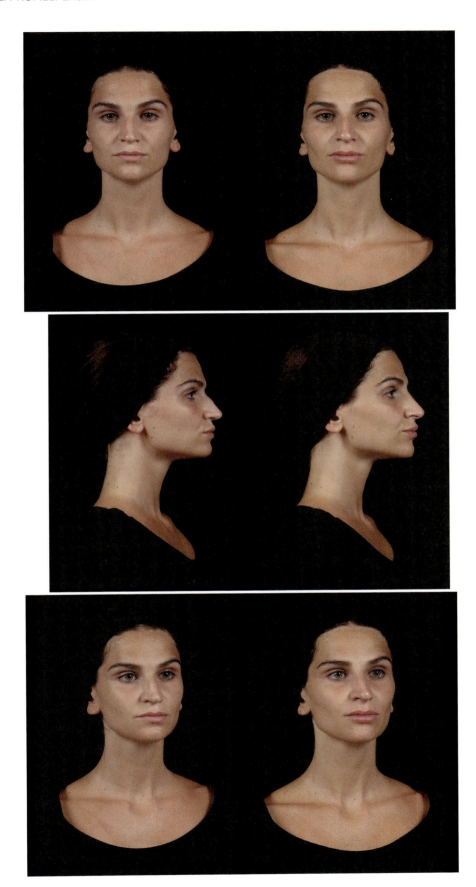

Figure 10.3.4 Patient 4: a, Frontal view, before and after; b, profile view, before and after; c, three-quarters view, before and after.

CHAPTER **10.4**

Clinical Case
The Slavic Face

Ekaterina Gutop

TREATMENT OF SURROUNDING AREAS: OPTICAL "CAMOUFLAGE"

The patient has typical characteristics of a Slavic face: light skin and eyes, oval shape of the face with soft features and sufficiently harmonious proportions. Despite their young age, the first signs of aging can be seen in the periorbital and zygomatic areas. A deficiency of volume in the superficial and deep fat compartments and a misbalance in proportions, with an accent on the lower face, create the perception of a tired and sad face. A lack of volume in bone structures increases this perception and is the target option for treatment with volumizer (Figure 10.4.1).

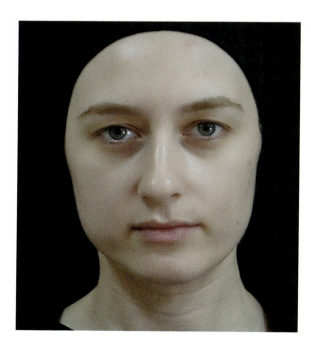

Figure 10.4.1 Before treatment.

Indications for correction with fillers are visible for the midface in the lateral and medial aspects, temporal, submalar, infraorbital areas and chin.

In spite of the presence of indications for a non-surgical rhinoplasty, harmonization by a full-face correction in surrounding areas with optical "camouflage" was selected for the patient. A natural appearance and feeling were maintained.

TREATMENT

The treatment was performed step by step in one session. The lateral parts of the face were treated first.

The deficiency of volume in the bone structure of the midface was corrected by deep injections of filler with high characteristics of elasticity and cohesivity for the lateral part of the zygomatic area with a cannula and fanning technique below the zygomatic ligament. Traction of soft tissues of the lateral part of the midface during injection is imperative to strengthen the effect of lifting, and the supraperiosteal plane of injection below the zygomatic ligament with a cannula helps to obtain an improvement not only in the treated area but also in surrounding zones. By using the insertion point for the cannula from the central part of the cheek, the correction of the submalar area was performed simultaneously.

The temporal area is a risky area and was injected as the next step by cannula. Smoothing the transition between the lateral part of the midface and temple was the goal for the injection. By using the insertion point for the cannula 1 cm below the zygomatic arch and pinching the tissues between the fingers of the other hand, sliding the cannula below the superficial temporal facia and smoothly injecting the filler by a fanning technique in an appropriate volume (less than 0.3 cc of the hyaluronic acid [HA] product), a visible aesthetical result was achieved. The midface and temples are the key areas for the harmony of the face as a whole.

Central facial zones such as the infraorbital, nasolabial, upper labial and lips were corrected as the next step

CLINICAL CASE: THE SLAVIC FACE

in the same session. The tear trough and dark circles were indications for treatment in the periorbital area. By correcting the midface and temples first, the problems of the periorbital zone became less visible and required less product for the direct approach.

Marking of the area between the lower orbital rim and lid cheek junction as a target zone for treatment should be done first. The author prefers correction of the infraorbital zone performed by cannula to minimize the risks of vessel complications. By injecting a low-hydrophilic HA filler below the orbicularis retaining ligament (ORL) in an appropriate amount (less than 0.3 cc) using a "microbolus" technique, correction of the lateral and medial part of the tear trough results in a fresh and natural appearance with less swelling.

The nasolabial fold was corrected with a cannula at the subcutaneous plane with a combination of bolus and fanning technique, with evident improvement not only in the treated area but also creating the optical illusion of lifting of the nose.

Lips are an important part of female facial attractiveness and harmony of the face. The anterior projection and improvement in shape and volume of the lower and upper lips were obtained by a delicate injection of filler to the superficial fat compartments of the upper and lower lip with a needle (Figures 10.4.2 and 10.4.3).

RESULT AND CONCLUSION

By treating the lateral zones of the face as the first step, not only the effect of lifting and harmonizing of the face as a whole was achieved, but an improvement of the central facial zones was visible. The orbital area, nasolabial fold and perioral area were treated next with a natural appearance and less product.

Non-surgical rhinoplasty was done indirectly by step-by-step injections in the surrounding area, which helped to create support and harmonize proportional relationships in parts of the face and achieved the effect of optical camouflage in the nasal area.

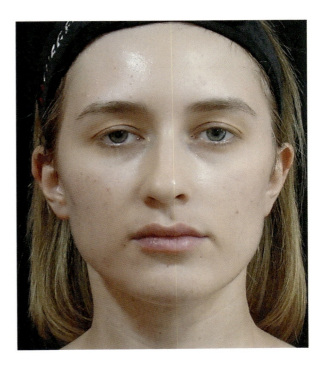

Figure 10.4.3 Treatment plan.

3 cc—Juvéderm Voluma—lateral part of the cheekbone—0.5 cc per side; 0.3 cc per side for the temples; 0.7 cc for submalar zone.

1 cc—Juvéderm Volux—chin with combination bolus and line-retrograde technique.

1 cc—Juvéderm Volbella 0.2 cc for the right and 0.3 for the left infraorbital area; 0.5 cc for perioral area.

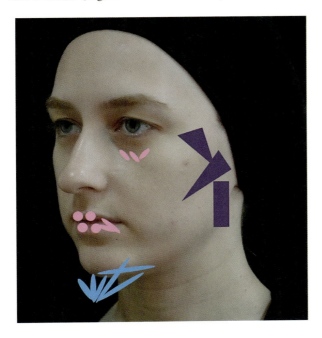

Figure 10.4.2 After treatment.

CHAPTER **10.5**

Clinical Case
Rhino 4-Point Technique with Fillers of Different Densities

Fernando Silikovich

This technique was developed 20 years ago. At that time, there were no cross-linked hyaluronic acid products; when they became available, the technique began to be modified and adapted until finally reaching the form described here. It has been performed on more than 23,000 patients, of whom 30% have had one or more surgical rhinoplasties. There have been nine accidental injections of hyaluronic acid intra-arterially that—with the hyaluronidase protocol used in the right time and form—have all resolved without necrosis of dermal tissue.

A 27G needle is required because, unlike the 30G needle, due to its size and the diameters of the nasal arteries, there is less possibility of intra-arterial injection. In addition, the concentration of hyaluronic acid used and its high G' is easier to handle with a 27G needle. Two types of hyaluronic acid are required, depending on the area of the nose to be treated. The dorsum of the nose requires a hyaluronic acid that we call "projective", with an intermediate G', a high G'', an intermediate E', and a high tau delta. In the columella, the hyaluronic acid required is what we call a "repositioner", with a high G', a low G', a high E', and a low tau delta. For this technique, the syringes of each product are used directly, without passing the product to other syringes. It is also required to have the necessary materials to activate a protocol for accidental injection of intra-arterial hyaluronic acid: 4–5 vials of hyaluronidase and a kit of adjuvants—aspirin 325 mg, prednisone 20 mg, and sildenafil or tadalafil 20 mg.

The Rhino 4-Point technique works on the nose in four zones: radix, nasion, tip, and columella. For the first three zones, projective hyaluronic acids are used, and for the last, repositioners. It works on the midline of the nose, in deep planes: supraperiostic, suprachondrial, and deep fat. Each time boluses are placed, they should not exceed 0.05 mL; if it is necessary to place more, the bolus should be repeated up to three times in different placements (Figures 10.5.1–10.5.2). In addition, prior to each bolus injection, aspiration should be carried out to confirm that it is not positive. With all these parameters, the risk of intra-arterial injection is considerably reduced. It is important to clarify that it is not always necessary to perform all four points or in a set order. In addition, we can also adapt the amounts of hyaluronic acid that we will place at each point to the aesthetic requirements of each case. The aesthetic design of each nose will be unique, and the technique will have to be adapted to each nose and not the other way around.

Point 1: With the non-injecting hand, both sides of the glabella are compressed, decreasing the flow of the dorsal artery of the nose. The injecting hand is positioned on the nasal midline in the most invaginated area of the radix. The syringe is at 70 degrees, and at the supraperiosteal layer, a bolus of 0.05 mL is placed. If necessary, the procedure can be repeated up to three times. Keep in mind that the idea is not to leave a Greek profile with the dorsum of the nose extremely straight, so you will always have to preserve a certain angularity.

Point 2: The non-injecting hand pinches the skin at the level of the nasion. Branches of the dorsal and lateral arteries of the nose are thus superficialized and, by placing a bolus of 0.025 mL in the supracondrial plane, the vascular risk is reduced. The syringe will also have an angle of 70 degrees. Note that in this area of the dorsum, the nasion, the skin is extremely thin, so, despite placing such a small bolus, you can sometimes notice overelevation of the skin. With light massage this overlifting can be corrected.

Point 3: The injecting hand is placed on the patient's forehead, generating an angle of 45 degrees. The syringe enters the interdomal space prior to the septum, direct to the middle of the columella, on the nasal midline, in deep fat. A bolus of 0.05 mL is placed first, then in retrograde injection another 0.05 mL, and finally, well on the upper interdomal space, a last bolus of 0.05 mL. During the placement of this last bolus the syringe is positioned at an angle of 70 degrees and

CLINICAL CASE: RHINO 4-POINT TECHNIQUE

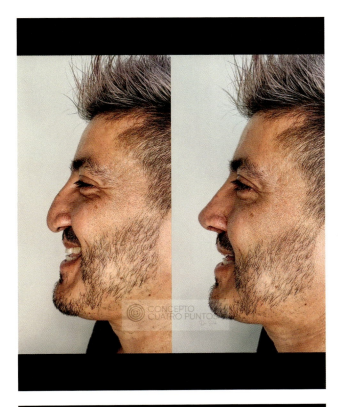

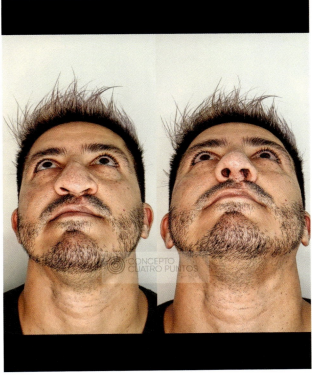

Figure 10.5.1 A male patient, 32 years old: Cleft palate and cleft lip with a history of 12 surgeries on the nose, palate and lip. Two different hyaluronic acids were used—one projective and another dense. At the tip of the nose 0.2 mL were placed intradomal, supraperiosteal, and midline; on the columella 0.15 mL were placed from the base to the tip midline in deep fat; in addition 0.15 mL were placed in the supraperiosteal nasal spine. In the piriform fossa 0.2 mL were placed, making a total of 0.9 mL of hyaluronic acid. The aesthetic effect lasted 12–18 months. In addition, the patient reported better ventilatory mechanics. (A) Profile view, before and after treatment; (B) inferior view, before and after treatment.

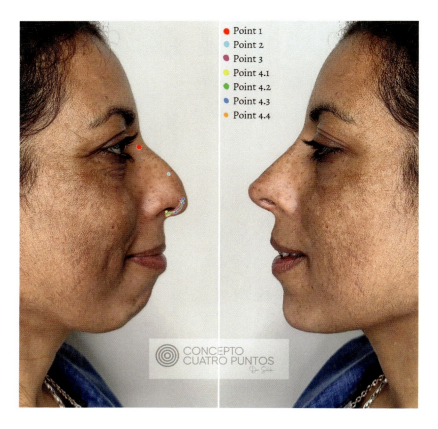

Figure 10.5.2 A female patient, 41 years old. (a) We used Merz Intense hyaluronic acid at points 1, 2, and 3 and Allergan Volume in points 4.1–4.4. Dosage was as follows: point 1, 0.05 mL supraperiosteal; point 2, 0.025 mL supraperiosteal; point 3, 0.05 mL in the intermediate columella, 0.05 mL retroinjection, and a 0.05-mL tip bolus; point 4.1, 0.05 mL nasal spine bolus; point 4.2 (entered in the columellar base) a 0.05 mL tip bolus, 0.05 retroinjection, and a last 0.05 mL base bolus; point 4.3 (entered in the columellar intermediate) as in point 4.2; point 4.4 (entered in the columellar base), one 0.05-mL bolus above and another 0.05-mL bolus on the columellar base. (b) Postoperative result.

the non-injecting hand compresses both domes. In this way this bolus can project the tip towards a more pyramidal and triangular shape.

Point 4: This point works on the columella with repositioning hyaluronic acids. It is subdivided into four more points.

Point 4.1: The syringe is placed on the midline at the base of the columella, at 90 degrees perpendicular to the nasal spine, and, supraperiosteally, a bolus of 0.05 mL is placed to open the nasolabial angle.

Point 4.2: This is the same entry point as for point 4.1 but the syringe is in a 10-degree position, resting on the chin. The needle is directed towards the tip and, in deep fat, a bolus of 0.05 mL is placed at the tip of the nose; then retroinjection also of 0.05 mL is performed. Finally there should be a last bolus of 0.05 mL at the base of the columella to give more rigidity and strength to the columella.

Point 4.3: This point is exactly the same as for point 4.2 with the difference that instead of entering the base of the columella, it enters the middle of it. It is also exactly the same as point 3 but with two differences: it is inverse to it (point 3 enters the tip of the nose and heads towards the middle of the columella, while point 4.3 enters the middle of the columella and heads towards the tip) and they use different types of hyaluronic acid (while point 3 uses projective hyaluronic acid to project and define triangularity of the tip, point 4.3 uses repositioner hyaluronic acid to raise the tip).

Point 4.4: This last point places two boluses of 0.05 mL, one on top of the other, at the base of the columella in deep fat to give more resistance and strength to the columella by preventing the tip of the nose from going down when smiling.

The average use of hyaluronic acid is 0.55 mL, with a minimum of 0.25 and a maximum of 1.05 mL. Often in the first 72 hours postoperatively there is mild edema, erythema, and pain that does not require the use of analgesia. It is recommended not to do physical activity in the first 48 hours, but the patient can resume their social and work activities immediately. Between weeks 5 and 7 in 20% of patients—mostly smokers and those who perform intense aerobic physical activity—part of the injected product is reabsorbed and requires reinjection. The results last between 12 months and up to more than 2 years, but it is advisable to repeat the procedure every 12 months to achieve a better and more lasting result.

Neither the Rhino 4-Point technique nor any other non-surgical rhinoplasty can replace a surgical rhinoplasty, and, obviously, not all cases are suitable. Clearly a substantial and indisputable difference is that surgery is a reducing technique and the use of hyaluronic acid is not. However, new global aesthetic trends are moving towards procedures that are less invasive, less complicated, and have less or no downtime; above all, these new trends are aimed towards balance and subtle harmony in the face and not so much toward irreversible radical transformation. The Rhino 4-Point technique offers that possibility and adapts perfectly to these new trends.

CHAPTER **10.6**

Clinical Case
Nasofrontal Angle with Ultrasound Correlation

Fernando Urdiales

There has been increasing use of hyaluronic acid (HA) for rhinomodulation as a solution for nose contour remodeling, principally at the nasofrontal angle and nasolabial angle. Lateral remodeling could be done with different techniques, but it should always use HA at different layers of the skin, applied at the supraperiosteal layer at the site of the angle and at the supracartilage location for lateral nose indications.

Cannulas are safer and more effective for all rhinomodulation treatments; needles could be used by advanced injectors. This is especially important in noses that have been operated on previously, as fibrosis and neovascularization are much more frequent in those cases.

We frequently use Voluma Lido and Volift. These are products with high viscoelasticity (G') and very low water retention; cohesivity is also very high with these products, and the integration is rapid and complete at the deep cellular subcutaneous tissue, supraperiosteal area, and supracartilage area as well. The volumes that we inject per session are variable, from 0.2 to 1.5 mL; we routinely conduct a touch-up session in 3–4 weeks. Treatment could last from 12 to 18 months in most patients (Figures 10.6.1–10.6.3).

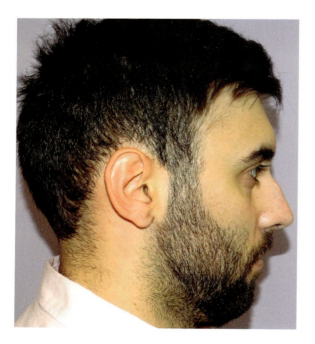 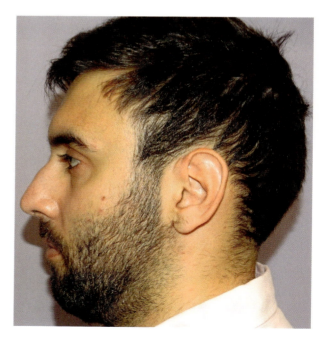

Figure 10.6.1 (a and b) The patient was a young man, 25 years old, with a nasofrontal angle of 143 degrees.

CLINICAL CASE: NASOFRONTAL ANGLE WITH ULTRASOUND CORRELATION

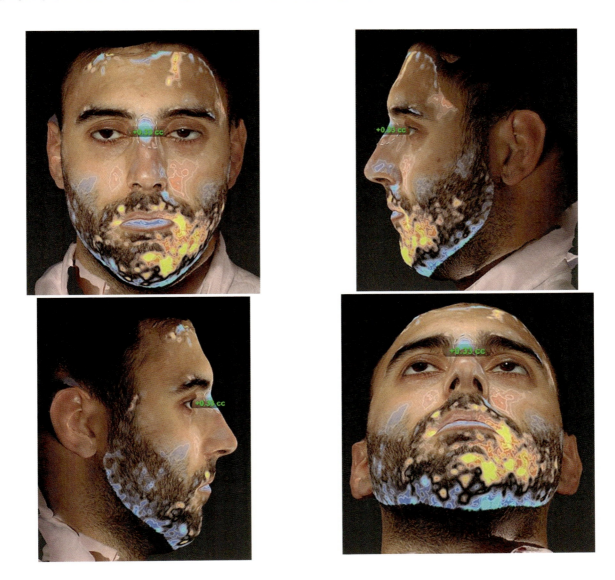

Figure 10.6.2 (a, b, c, d) One session of Voluma Lido HA with a 27G cannula, using the supraperiostic bolus-fanning technique.

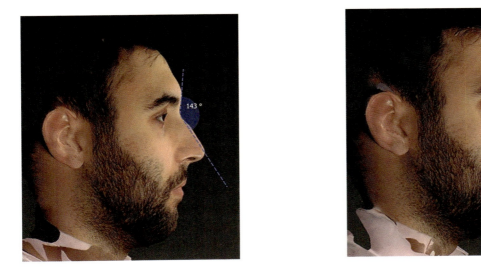

Figure 10.6.3 (a and b) The result obtained was an 8-degree increase (to 151 degrees) in the nasofrontal angle.

Ultrasound is a useful tool to help make a diagnosis of the different reabsorbable and permanent fillers in the face, because different fillers have different echographic patterns. As we have shown elsewhere [ref 1], four patterns can be identified:

1. A globular pattern shows an anechoic image with posterior echogenic reinforcement. This is typical immediately after HA injection in the area (Figure 10.6.4).
2. A snow grain pattern is typical in silicon oil fillers (the small snow grain pattern) or in calcium hydroxylapatite fillers (the coarse snow grain pattern). This presents as a hyperechogenic image with echogenic posterior shadow (silicon).
3. A heterogeneous pattern is the typical pattern of healthy skin with hypoechoic and hyperechoic images and is the pattern of HA integrated with skin.

The best ultrasound to use in aesthetic medicine must have more than 12 Mhz of emission frequency, using a linear probe.

REFERENCE

1. Fernando Urdiales-Gálvez F, De cabo-Francés F, Bové I. Ultrasound patterns of different dermal filler materials used in aesthetics. J Cosmet Dermatol. 2021;00:1–8.

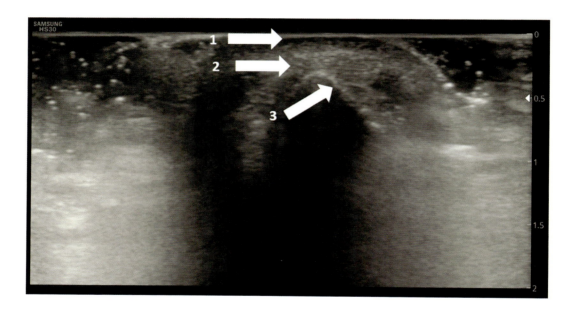

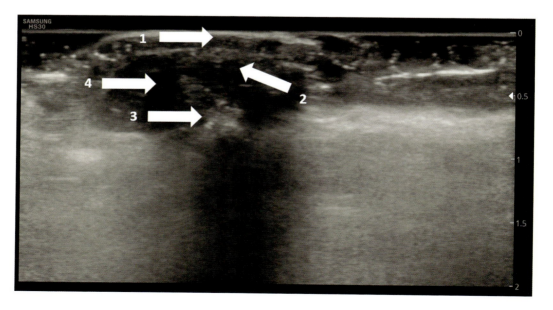

Figure 10.6.4 Ultrasound imaging: (a) before—1, epidermis; 2, subcutaneous fat; 3, nasal bone; (b) after—1, epidermis; 2, subcutaneous fat; 3, nasal bone; 4, globular HA ultrasound pattern (anechoic).

CHAPTER **10.7**

My Tinkerbell Tip Lift Technique

K. Kay Durairaj

INTRODUCTION

As a nasal surgeon, my understanding of nasal proportions and anatomy has allowed me to use surgical analytics in the setting of non-surgical rhinoplasty techniques. My philosophy towards non-surgical rhinoplasties is to place filler with the utmost precision and surgical knowledge of anatomy. The filler should be used in a similar fashion to a surgical cartilage graft. The most important aspects of obtaining precise results with liquid rhinoplasties are the filler depth placement, the plane of placement, and the controlled amounts used. Microdroplet quantities are used to effectively prevent excess swelling of the nose and reduce the possibility of a bloated or puffy appearance. Maintaining very small microdroplets is important to preserve a sharper and more precise result. Aspiration is performed with each injection. The injector who is undertaking liquid rhinoplasties needs to master nasal anatomy at the level of a surgeon. The filler should be placed whenever possible in the plane of the periosteum and perichondrium, and it will be safest and most avascular by staying directly in the midline. With this precise technique, our patients have a high satisfaction rate and minimal downtime while achieving elegant refinement of primary contour irregularities, posttraumatic, and postsurgical rhinoplasty corrections.

CASE 1

A 32-year-old male (see Figure 10.7.1) patient presented with complaints of difficulty breathing through the nose and severe nasal congestion. The patient underwent surgical septoplasty in 2016. The patient was successfully treated and had correction of a deviated septum and septal spur. His immediate postoperative course was uneventful. Subsequently, two years following his nasal procedure, the patient complained of a new-onset, moderately severe depression in the bridge of the nose. He denied any history of nasal trauma and felt that he had gradual shifting and change in the nasal dorsum. His physical exam showed an upper dorsal hump deformity and mid-dorsal saddle deformity. A subsequent computed tomography (CT) scan of the sinuses showed normal sinuses with a deficiency of his septal cartilage. The patient was given the option to undergo surgery to correct the defect with an autologous dorsal auricular draft vs. injectable filler. He elected to have injectable filler placed on the dorsal of the nose with the desired goal to fix the dorsal hump deformity, drooping tip, and saddle nose deformity.

TECHNIQUE

The patient's nose was sterilized with betadine externally, and internal nostrils were also sterilized with betadine. Topical lidocaine/tetracaine 23%/7% numbing cream was applied to the nasal dorsum for 20 minutes. The nose was then cleansed with alcohol and photographs were documented. The patient was given a detailed informed consent discussion that explained all the risks, benefits, and alternatives to non-surgical rhinoplasty. The risks included bleeding, infection, vascular necrosis, skin necrosis, extremely rare risk of blindness, and/or loss of vision. After careful measurement of his nasal anatomy, he was injected with 0.5 ccs of medium-density hyaluronic acid filler, concentration of 20 mg/mL with 0.3% lidocaine, with a G' of 531 made by Galderma using a 29-gauge needle.

The first bolus of injection was inserted at the radix and directly on the periosteum in the midline. While stabilizing the needle, the area was aspirated with a BD insulin syringe. A 0.05-cc volume at each injection point was used. The nasal dorsal saddle nose defect was palpated and corrected. A retrograde linear injection technique was used. Supraperiosteal injections were performed while staying directly in the midline at the glabellar nasion area,

DOI: 10.1201/9781003304623-31

and deep dermal injections were performed in the area of the nasal alae and tip. After injecting the radix, the rhinion was injected to match the height of the nasal hump. It is my preference to adjust the height of the hump first. Then, the tip height was adjusted and lifted proportionally. In constructing the nasal tip, I use filler in a similar configuration to a tip shield graft. Tip shield grafts are used in rhinoplasty when tip sutures are not enough and are an effective way to increase tip definition, fill defects, and shape the tip. Filler was gradually built up in layers in the shape of a pyramid configuration at the nasal tip. The serial puncture injection technique should be followed for the nasal tip to prevent the creation of a bulbous nose.

Skin thickness is assessed during the injection. Thick skin with large sebaceous glands and pore size may prevent the creation of sharp definition with non-surgical rhinoplasties. This patient had thin skin, and it was possible to configure the shape of the nasal tip to improve the projection. Filler collapses and tends to flatten when people have very active nasalis muscles. To prevent this from occurring, 4 units of toxin were administered at the base of the nose. Pre- and postoperative substantial changes were achieved, with change in the nasolabial angle from 60 degrees to 90 degrees, the nasofacial angle from 40 degrees to 45 degrees, and the nasofrontal angle from 120 degrees to 125 degrees. The correction of the saddle nose was improved by 3–4 mm to give a straight nasal dorsum. The patient was very satisfied with the results, and results lasted 2–3 years following treatment.

CASE 2

A 38-year-old female (Figure 10.7.2) presented with a dorsal hump deformity and drooping tip desiring a non-surgical rhinoplasty. Treatment was carried out with 0.5 cc of medium-density hyaluronic acid filler concentration of 20 mg/mL with 0.3% lidocaine, with a G' of 531, made by Galderma, injected using a 29-gauge 5-mm needle on an insulin syringe. The patient reported high satisfaction with the results. One month later, the patient received 0.2 cc in the nasal tip and bridge. On September 16, 2020, the patient returned for a touch-up and received an additional 0.2 cc. The patient showed subsequent sustained improvements. The patient received an additional 0.4 cc on November 2, 2020; July 1, 2021; and October 14, 2021, for her subsequent touch-up visits.

TECHNIQUES

The first bolus of injection was inserted directly on the periosteum. It is advised to occlude the dorsal nasal arteries while injecting in the rare occasion that filler may

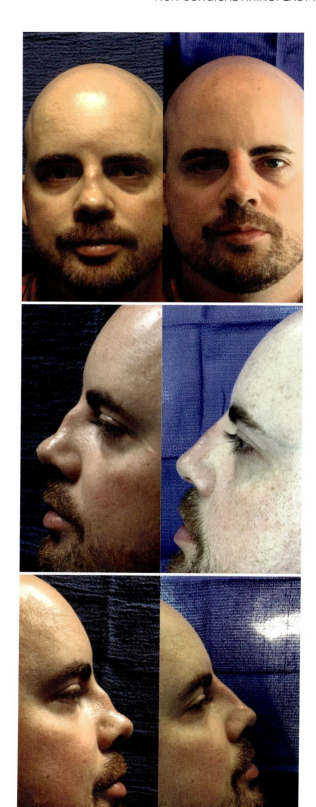

Figure 10.7.1 Case 1 patient

migrate. Increments of 0.05 cc were injected into the radix and at vertical columns of height to increase the dorsal nasofrontal angle and improve inadequate nasal projection. To correct the patient's drooping tip, the needle was inserted perpendicular upwards at a 45-degree angle. The patient demonstrated excellent improvements post-treatment, with a change in the nasolabial angle from 85 degrees to 105 degrees, in the nasofacial angle from 30 degrees to 35 degrees, and in the nasofrontal angle from 130 degrees to 125 degrees.

CONCLUSION

Dramatic change can be achieved with a non-surgical rhinoplasty. These case studies demonstrate my Tinkerbell tip lift techniques used to correct a dorsal hump, saddle nose, asymmetry, and drooping tips with the vision of using dermal filler as a sculpting agent. In 2019, 207 liquid rhinoplasty procedures were performed in my practice. The number of patients who returned for a second treatment one year later was 56. Most patients have filler duration of 12–18 months. The likelihood of patients repeating the procedure was 98.2%. The median reported pain level on a scale of 1–10 was ranked 2. The overall patient satisfaction rate was very high. Non-surgical rhinoplasty is a safe and effective technique to improve the appearance of the nose.

BIBLIOGRAPHY

1. Bertossi D, Magagnotto N, Chirumbolo S, D'Souza A, Nocini R. Nonsurgical rhinoplasty: Long-term follow-up of high G' HA nasal injections. Facial Plast Surg. 2022 Feb 14. doi: 10.1055/s-0042–1742431. Epub ahead of print. PMID: 35158387.
2. Bertossi D, Malchiodi L, Albanese M, Nocini R, Nocini P. Nonsurgical rhinoplasty with the novel hyaluronic acid filler VYC-25L: results using a nasal grid approach. Aesthet Surg J. 2021;41(6):NP512–NP520.
3. Kurkjian TJ, Ahmad J, Rohrich RJ. Soft-tissue fillers in rhinoplasty. Plast Reconstr Surg. 2014;133(2):121e–126e.
4. Redaelli A. Medical rhinoplasty with hyaluronic acid and botulinum toxin A: a very simple and quite effective technique. J Cosmet Dermatol. 2008;7(3):210–220.

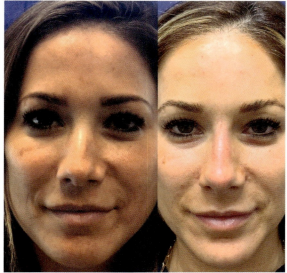
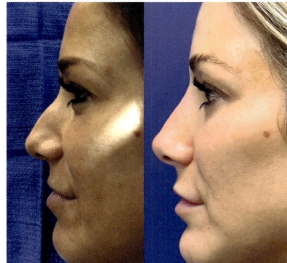
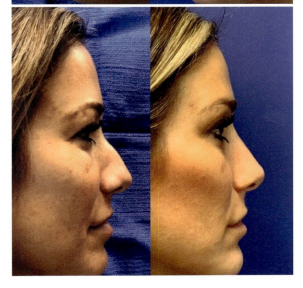

Figure 10.7.2 Case 2 patient

CHAPTER **10.8**

Clinical Case
Long Duration of HA Fillers in the Nose

Per Heden

Non-surgical options are very useful in some cases where the surgical option is not (yet) acceptable to the patient; the results can have long duration.

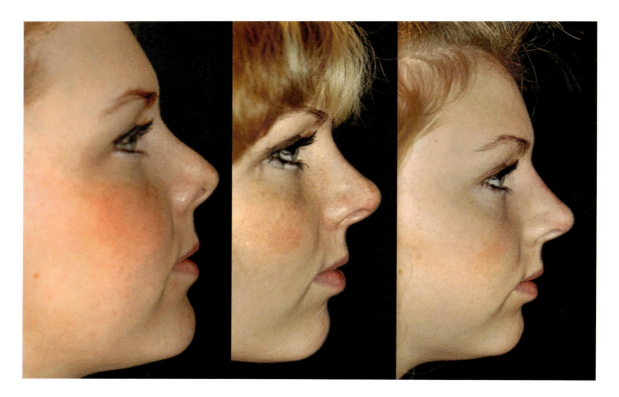

Figure 10.8.1 The patient was a young girl concerned about a short nose who wanted to avoid surgery if possible. (a) Before treatment with HA injection. With a 25G cannula 0.2 mL were injected along the dorsum and 0.3 mL in the columella and distal tip. Another 0.2 mL were injected intradermally with a needle to provide better tip projection. (b) At follow-up 3 months later, before secondary injection with a similar volume in the same locations. (c) Six months after the first injection

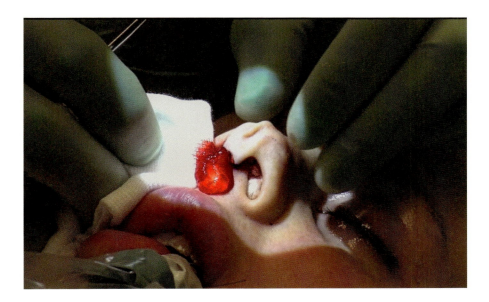

Figure 10.8.2 Four years later the patient requested converting the non-surgical nasal reshaping to a permanent surgical result. At an open rhinoplasty a large amount of HA (estimated to be two-thirds of the injected volume, although it was not possible to measure exactly) still remained in the nose, despite the long duration since the last injection (see also Video 10.8.1. Available at https://resourcecentre.routledge.com/books/9781032303444).

CHAPTER **10.9**

Clinical Case
Nasal Hump (Multiple Approach)

Philippe Magistretti

This female patient presented with a nasal hump, with thick skin. I injected her on the nasal base and then on the anterior nasal spine with Volux (Allergan-Abbvie, USA), then on the infratip lobule, as well as on the nasal tip between the domes, and finally on the glabella (0.2 mL) and the nasal dorsum (0.2 mL).

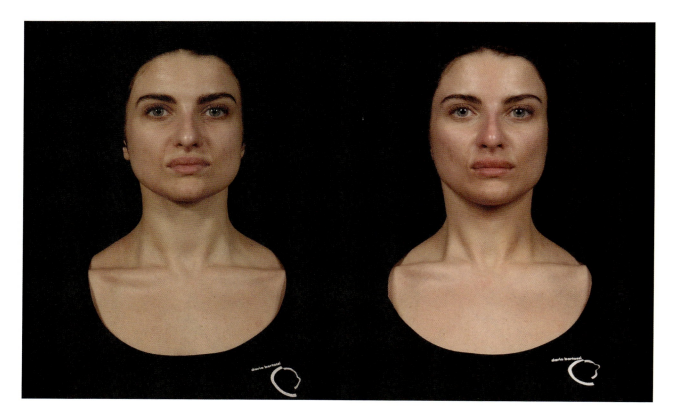

Figure 10.9.1 Frontal view, before and after.

CLINICAL CASE: NASAL HUMP (MULTIPLE APPROACH)

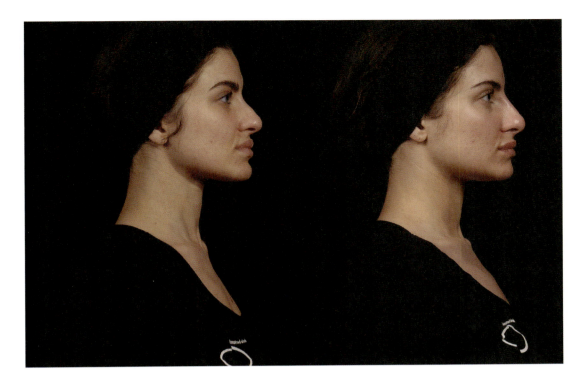

Figure 10.9.2 Profile view, before and after.

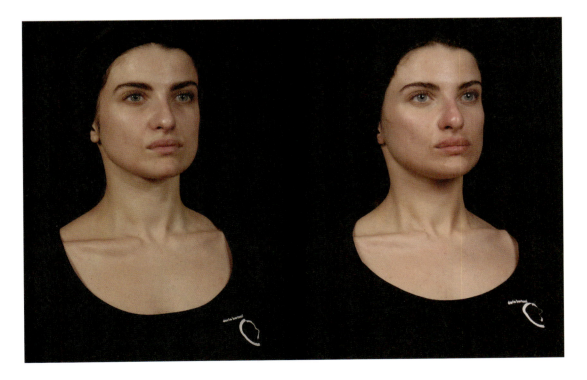

Figure 10.9.3 Three-quarters view, before and after.

CHAPTER **10.10**

Clinical Case
Nasal Hump (Dorsum Approach)

Rami Abadi

Hyaluronic acid fillers may be used to correct the shape of the nose and improve an uneven hump, correct imperfections, and help lift the tip of the nose. It is a fast procedure that requires minimal downtime and can have a great impact on the patient's self-perception and confidence. The results last between 12 and 18 months.

The patient was a 30-year-old lady complaining of a hump on her nose and concerned about her profile view. She requested a non-surgical modality to correct her imperfection. She was injected on the dorsum of the nose using Juvéderm Voluma 0.3 mL via a 27G needle deep down to the bone. We can see the smoothening of the dorsal hump and improvement in her profile view (Figure 10.10.1).

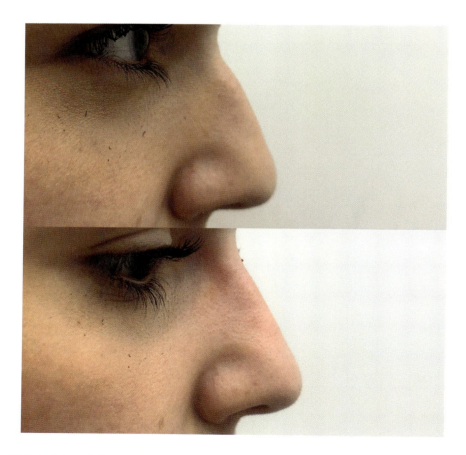

Figure 10.10.1 (A) Before non-surgical rhinoplasty; (B) after non-surgical rhinoplasty.

CHAPTER **10.11**

Clinical Case
Rhino-Modeling in South America

Raúl Banegas

The southern region of America has had a lot of immigration influence from different parts of the world, depending on the time and depending on the country. For example, in Brazil, the influence of Africans has been especially relevant, causing the mixture of ethnic groups to produce a special type of face: the "mestizo" or "mulatto". Some regions of Central America and the Caribbean have had a similar imprint. If we go farther south, both Argentina and Chile have not been influenced by African ethnicity, but rather European and Middle Eastern, in some cases mixed with natives. Therefore, the result varies a lot depending on the country of South America that we are analyzing.

The more mestizo or negroid influence the population has, the more we will have to take into account nasal filling as "nasal augmentation" techniques, both in projection of the dorsum and in the nasal tip. The main characteristic of the mestizo nose is the flattening of the back in the profile view, but also its widening in the frontal view (see Video 10.11.1. Available at https://resourcecentre.routledge.com/books/9781032303444).

If we evaluate the different anatomical parts, we can divide the nose into the radix (nasofrontal angle), dorsum, tip, and columellar regions.

Radix: The injection must be done by clamping the soft tissue to raise as many vessels as possible and leave the product at the supraperiosteal level. It should be noted that the largest depression should be located at the height of the tarsal fold.

Dorsum: I recommend doing the injection with a needle, entering perpendicular to the skin and leaving microboluses on the entire back. In this way, the elevation of the skin will be much more noticeable than when it is done with a cannula, parallel to the skin.

Tip: In the case of poorly projecting tips, it is necessary to enter between both alar cartilages and reach the nasal spine, passing through the lower edge of the nasal septum, and make a significant pillar (0.4 mL on average) to achieve a significant projection.

Columella: The nasolabial angle should be between 95 and 105 degrees and the columella below the nasal wing between 3 and 5 mm. Only inject into the nasal spine if you need to increase the angle; otherwise, it should not be injected in that area.

Defining the nasal tip: The domes of both alar cartilages should be defined. To do this, each dome is approached from the side, and the aim is to reach the desired place with the tip of the needle. The product is left between the skin and the cartilage. It should never be injected intradermally.

The product to be used must have a high G' in order to achieve the goal of moving the nose away from the face. The average product used is 1 mL, although sometimes this amount can be exceeded. Personally, I use Juvéderm Voluma, Juvéderm Volux, or Juvéderm Ultra 4 (Ultra Plus). See Figure 10.11.1.

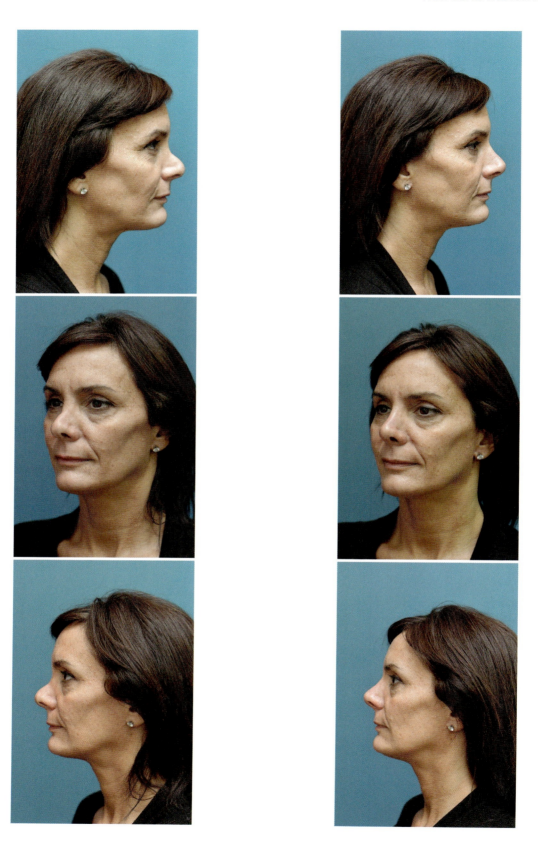

Figure 10.11.1 A 43-year-old woman with three previous surgeries. Both triangular cartilages collapsed due to an overresection, and there is a similar situation in the septum and crus lateralis of both alars, with consequent ventilatory insufficiency: (a-c) before and (d-f) after rhino-modeling.

Video 10.11.1 Evaluation of a 34-year-old patient with "mestizo" nose and lack of support in the nasal tip. Available at https://resourcecentre.routledge.com/books/9781032303444

Index

Note: Page numbers in *italic* indicate a figure or diagram and page numbers in **bold** indicate a table on the corresponding page.

A

acne, 59–60, *59–60*, **61**, 71–72
    OCT, and, 71
    RCM, and, 72
aesthetic treatments, *see* nasal aesthetic treatments
alar retraction or collapse, 97
anatomy
    deep anatomy, 27–30
        bone, 30, *30*
        cartilage, 30–31, *30–31*
        fat, 27–28, *28*
        innervation, 29, *29–30*
        muscles, 28–29, *28*
        skin, 27, *27*
        vascularization, 29, *29*
    surface anatomy, 21–24
        introduction, 21
        lines identifying specific points, 24, *24*
        nasal grid, 24, *24*
        nasal surrounding areas, 23, *23*
        nasal terminology, 21–23, *22*
Asian cases, 139–141, *140–141*
assessment, *see* preoperative diagnosis
autoimmune diseases
    RCM, and, 75

B

basal cell carcinoma (BCC), 64–66, *64–66*
bone, 30, *30*
botulinum toxin, 7–8
    bunny lines, 7–8, 100
    market, 13
    sagging nasal tip, 8, 100
    statistical analysis on treated patients and stability of filler, 100
bunny lines
    botulinum toxin, 7–8, 100

C

"camouflage," optical, 147
cartilage, 30–31, *30–31*
cheek and zygomatic arch 110–111
clinical aspects
    clinical defects and the technical approach
        equipment, 39, *39*
        framing technique, 39–40
        patient preparation, 39
        picture protocol, 40, *40–44*
        technical devices, introduction to, 35–39, *36–38*
    patient consultation, 45–46, *45*
        MD Codes, 46–47, *47*
clinical cases
    Asian cases, 139–141, *140–141*
    long duration of HA fillers in the nose, 161–162, *161–162*
    nasal hump
        dorsum approach, 165, *166*
        multiple approach, 163–164, *163–164*
    nasofrontal angle with ultrasound correlation, 153–155, *153–155*
    non-surgical rhinoplasty, 101–107, *102–107*
        long-term correction after five years, 135, *135–138*
    profileplasty, 143–146, *143–146*
    rhino 4-point technique with fillers of different densities, 149–152, *150–151*
    rhino-modeling in South America, 167, *168*
    Slavic cases, 147–148, *147–148*
    surgical rhinoplasty, 82–84, *82–84*
    tinkerbell tip lift technique, 157–159, *158–159*
clinical defects and the technical approach
    equipment, 39, *39*
    framing technique, 39–40
    patient preparation, 39
    picture protocol, 40, *40–44*
    technical devices, introduction to, 35–39, *36–38*
closed nasal labial angle nasal base retrusion, 90
combined devices, 9
complications, 121–128, *122–123*, *125*, **126**, *127*
    classification of, 124–125
    diagnosis and therapy of, 125–127
        late occurring reactions, 126–127
        vascular complications, 125–126
    prevention, 122–124
computed tomography (CT), 75
consultation, patient, 45–46, *45*
    MD Codes, 46–47, *47*
crooked nose deformity, 96
CT, *see* computed tomography

D

deep anatomy, 27–30, *see also* anatomy
    bone, 30, *30*
    cartilage, 30–31, *30–31*
    fat, 27–28, *28*
    innervation, 29, *29–30*
    muscles, 28–29, *28*
    skin, 27, *27*
    vascularization, 29, *29*
deep glabella, 94
defects, clinical, *see* clinical defects and the technical approach
dependent tip, 91
dermatitis, 62, *62*
dermoscopy, 69
    impetigo, and, 72
    lichen planus, and, 73
    psoriasis, and, 73
    rosacea, and, 70
    seborrheic dermatitis, and, 72
deviated nose, 95
devices, *see* technical devices
diagnosis, *see* complications; preoperative diagnosis
D-OCT, *see* speckle-variance OCT
dynamic OCT, *see* speckle-variance OCT

E

endoscopic diagnosis and instrumentation tools, 54
ethnic features, 86–87, *86–87*, *see also* Asian cases; Slavic cases
    leptorrhine nose, 87, *87*
    mesorrhine nose, 86, *86*
    platyrrhine nose, 86, *86*
equipment, 39, *39*

F

fat, 27–28, *28*
fibrous papule (FP), 63, *63*
framing technique, 39–40

G

grid, nasal, 24, *24*

H

HA *see* hyaluronic acid (HA) fillers
herpes simplex virus (HSV), 58, *59*, 70–71
    dermoscopy, and, 71
    LC-OCT, and, 71
    RCM, and, 71
hidden columella nasal base retrusion 89
hyaluronic acid (HA) fillers, 3–4, *see also* non-surgical profileplasty; non-surgical rhinoplasty
    complications, 121–128, *122–123*, *125*, **126**, *127*
    market, 11–12

I

impetigo 59, 72–72
    dermoscopy, and, 72
    RCM, and, 72
infective/inflammatory conditions, 58
inflammatory conditions, *see* infective/inflammatory conditions
injectable profileplasty, 115–116
injection plan and procedure, 97–99
innervation, 29, *29–30*

L

late occurring reactions, 126–127, *see also* complications
LC-OCT, *see* line-field confocal optical coherence tomography

leptorrhine nose, 87, *87*
lichen planus, 73
    dermoscopy, and, 73
    OCT, and, 74
    RCM, and, 74
line-field confocal optical coherence tomography (LC-OCT), 69
    active herpes infection, 71
lines identifying specific points, 24, *24*
lips, 112–113
long duration of HA fillers in the nose, 161–162, *161–162*

M

magnetic resonance imaging (MRI), 52–53, *52*
malignant melanoma (MM), 66–67, *67*
market
    botulinum toxin, 13
    hyaluronic acid (HA) fillers, 11–12
MD Codes, 46–47, *47*
mesorrhine nose, 86, *86*
muscles, 28–29, *28*

N

nasal aesthetic treatments
    botulinum toxin, 7–8
        bunny lines, 7–8
        market, 13
        sagging nasal tip, 8
    combined devices, 9
    hyaluronic acid (HA) fillers, 3–4
        market, 11–12
    introduction, 1
    social networks, impact of, 15–17
nasal base retrusion, 89
nasal boundaries, 87, *87*
nasal grid, 24, *24*, 87
nasal hump, 92
    clinical cases, 163–164, *163–164*, 165, *166*
nasal surrounding areas, 23, *23*
nasal terminology, 21–23, *22*
nasolabial region, 111–112
nasofrontal angle with ultrasound correlation, 153–155, *153–155*
non-melanoma skin cancer (NMSC), 64, **65**
non-surgical profileplasty, 115–118, *116*, see *also* clinical cases
    injectable, 115–116
    introduction, 115
    surgical profileplasty, and, 116–118
non-surgical rhinoplasty, 85–101, see *also* clinical cases
    ethnic features, 86–87, *86–87*
    practical approaches, 87–101, *87–100*
        alar retraction or collapse, 97
        assessment, 88
        bunny lines, 100
        closed nasal labial angle nasal base retrusion, 90
        crooked nose deformity, 96
        deep glabella, 94
        dependent tip, 91
        deviated nose, 95
        hidden columella nasal base retrusion, 89
        injection plan and procedure, 97–99
        nasal base retrusion, 89
        nasal hump, 92
        overprojected nose, 94
        results, 100
        saddle nose, 93
        sagging nasal tip, 100
        secondary defects, 96
        statistical analysis on treated patients and stability of filler, 100
    introduction, 85–86
    nasal boundaries, 87, *87*
    posttreatment, 101

O

OCT, see optical coherence tomography
optical "camouflage," 147
optical coherence tomography (OCT), 69
    acne, and, 71
    lichen planus, and, 74
    psoriasis, and, 74
    seborrheic dermatitis, and, 72–73
overprojected nose, 94

P

patient consultation, 45–46, *45*
    MD Codes, 46–47, *47*
patient preparation, 39
perioral dermatitis, 61, *61*
picture protocol, 40, *40–44*
platyrrhine nose, 86, *86*
points
    lines identifying specific points, 24, *24*
posttreatment, 101
preoperative diagnosis and assessment, 51–75, 88
    endoscopic diagnosis and instrumentation tools, 54
    introduction, 51
    magnetic resonance imaging (MRI), 52–53, *52–53*
    other techniques, 55
    skin conditions affecting the nose and perinasal area, 57–67
        acne, 59–60, *59–60*, **61**, 71–72
        autoimmune diseases, 75
        basal cell carcinoma, (BCC), 64–66, *65*
        conditions mandating pretreatment before filler procedures, 58
        dermatitis, 62, *62*
        fibrous papule (FP), 63, *63*
        herpes simplex virus (HSV), 58, *59*, 70–71
        impetigo, 59, 72
        infective/inflammatory conditions, 58
        introduction, 57–58, **58**
        lichen planus, 73–74
        lupus, *74*
        malignant melanoma (MM), 66–66
        non-melanoma skin cancer (NMSC), 64, **65**
        perioral dermatitis (POD), 61, *61*
        psoriasis, 73–74, *74*
        rosacea 60–61, *60*, **61**, 70
        scleroderma, *75*
        sebaceous hyperplasia (SH), 63
        seborrheic dermatitis (SD), 63, 72–73
        seborrheic keratoses (SK), 63–64, *64*
    tools, 69–75
        computed tomography (CT), 75
        dermoscopy, 69–74
        line-field confocal optical coherence tomography (LC-OCT), 69, 71
        optical coherence tomography (OCT), 69, 71–74
        reflectance confocal microscopy (RCM), 69–75
        speckle-variance OCT (dynamic OCT; D-OCT), 69–70
        ultrasound techniques, 53–54, *53*
preparation, patient, 39
prevention of severe complications, 122–124
profileplasty, see non-surgical profileplasty
protocol, picture, 40, *40–44*
psoriasis, 73
    dermoscopy, and, 73
    OCT, and, 74
    RCM, and, 74

R

RCM, see reflectance confocal microscopy
reflectance confocal microscopy (RCM), 69–70
    acne, and, 71
    autoimmune diseases, 75
    impetigo, and, 72
    lichen planus, and, 74
    psoriasis, and, 74
    rosacea, and, 70
    seborrheic dermatitis, and, 73
rhino 4-point technique with fillers of different densities, 149–152, *150–151*
rhinoplasty, see non-surgical rhinoplasty; surgical rhinoplasty
rosacea, 60–61, *60*, **61**, 70
    dermoscopy, and, 70
    D-OCT, and, 70
    RCM, and, 70

S

saddle nose, 93
sagging nasal tip
    botulinum toxin, 8, 100
sebaceous hyperplasia, 63
seborrheic dermatitis (SD), 63, 72–73
    dermoscopy, and, 72
    OCT, and, 72–73
    RCM, and, 73
seborrheic keratoses (SK), 63–64, *64*
secondary defects, 96
skin, 27, *27*
skin conditions affecting the nose and perinasal area, 57–67
    acne, 59–60, *59–60*, **61**, 71–72
    autoimmune diseases, 75

INDEX

basal cell carcinoma, (BCC), 64–66, *65*
conditions mandating pretreatment before filler procedures, 58
dermatitis, 62, *62*
fibrous papule (FP), 63, *63*
herpes simplex virus (HSV), 58, *59*, 70–71
impetigo, 59, 72
infective/inflammatory conditions, 58
introduction, 57–58, **58**
lichen planus, 73–74
lupus, *74*
malignant melanoma (MM), 66–66
non-melanoma skin cancer (NMSC), 64, **65**
perioral dermatitis (POD), 61, *61*
psoriasis, 73–74, *74*
rosacea 60–61, *60*, **61**, 70
scleroderma, *75*
sebaceous hyperplasia (SH), 63
seborrheic dermatitis (SD), 63, 72–73
seborrheic keratoses (SK), 63–64, *64*
Slavic cases, 147–148, *147–148*
social networks
    impact of, 15–17
speckle-variance OCT (dynamic OCT; D-OCT), 69
    rosacea, and, 70

stability of filler, 100
statistical analysis on treated patients and stability of filler, 100
surface anatomy, 21–24
    introduction, 21
    lines identifying specific points, 24, *24*
    nasal grid, 24, *24*
    nasal surrounding areas, 23, *23*
    nasal terminology, 21–23, *22*
surgical profileplasty, 116–118
surgical rhinoplasty, 79–84
    clinical case, 82–84, *82–84*
    surgical technique, 79–82, *80–82*
surrounding areas, nasal, 23, *23*, 109–113, *109*
    cheek and zygomatic arch 110–111
    introduction, 109
    lips, 112–113
    nasolabial region, 111–112
    Slavic cases, 147

T

technical approach, *see* clinical defects and the technical approach
technical devices
    introduction to, 35–39, *36–38*
    technique, surgical 79–82, *80–82*
    terminology, nasal, 21–23, *22*
    therapy of complications, 125–127
        late occurring reactions, 126–127
        vascular complications, 125–126
tinkerbell tip lift technique, 157–159, *158–159*
treatments, *see* nasal aesthetic treatments

U

ultrasound techniques, 53–54, *53*
    nasofrontal angle with ultrasound correlation, 153–155, *153–155*

V

vascular complications, 125–126, *see also* complications
vascularization, 29, *29*

Z

zygomatic arch 110–111

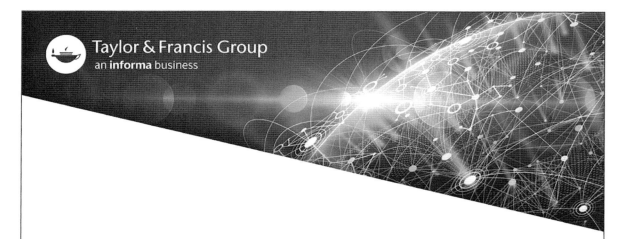